Dancing on Quicksand

Dancing on Quicksand

A Gift of Friendship
in the Age of Alzheimer's

Marilyn Mitchell

Johnson Books
BOULDER

Published by Johnson Books, a division of Johnson Publishing Company, 1880 South 57th Court, Boulder, Colorado 80301. E-mail: books@jpcolorado.com.

9 8 7 6 5 4 3 2

Cover design by Debra B. Topping
Cover photograph of David Touff at his daughter's wedding in 1972, courtesy of the Touff family

Library of Congress Cataloging-in-Publication Data
Mitchell, Marilyn, 1945–
    Dancing on quicksand: a gift of friendship in the age of Alzheimer's / Marilyn Mitchell
        p. ; cm.
    ISBN 1-55566-321-4 (alk. paper)
    1. Touff, David, 1905– —Health. 2. Mitchell, Marilyn, 1945–
3. Alzheimer's disease—Patients—United States—Biography. 4. Caregivers—United States—Biography.
    [DNLM: 1. Touff, David, 1905– 2. Mitchell, Marilyn, 1945– 3. Alzheimer Disease—rehabilitation—Personal Narratives. 4. Alzheimer Disease—rehabilitation—Popular Works. 5. Activities of Daily Living—Personal Narratives. 6. Activities of Daily Living—Popular Works. 7. Caregivers—Personal Narratives. 8. Caregivers—Popular Works. 9. Dementia—rehabilitation—Personal Narratives. 10. Dementia—rehabilitation—Popular Works. WT 155 M682d 2002] I. Title.
    RC523.T62 M55 2002
    362.1'96831'0092—dc21

2002000940

Printed in the United States by
Johnson Printing
1880 South 57th Court
Boulder, Colorado 80301

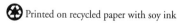 Printed on recycled paper with soy ink

For My Parents,
Bea and Bill Mitchell,
neither of whom was educated
beyond high school.
My mother, a preacher's daughter,
bright, creative, and articulate,
who gave me an appreciation
for the power of words.

My father, a farmer's son,
a man of immense compassion
who taught me,
whether dealing with animals or people,
"Always try to see the situation
from the other guy's perspective.
Remember, all behavior is caused.
The fox won't bite you
because he's bad;
he'll bite you because he's afraid."

It astonishes me
that having faced the terror,
we continue to live,
even to live
with a great deal of joy.*

—Alice Trillin, 1938–2001
College professor, author, producer of award-winning
art and educational documentaries

IN HER BOOK *Dear Bruno*, a letter written to a boy with cancer, the late Alice Trillin cautioned readers not to "make the mistake of thinking that knights who talk 'brave talk' and make jokes about dragons don't understand how truly dangerous dragons are." Ms. Trillin, herself a survivor of cancer, suggested, "The bravest knights, having fought the fiercest battles, understand the nature of dragons better than anyone."**

Attempting to sugarcoat dementia would be an affront to the millions who have experienced its horror and heartbreak. If there is humor, even occasionally a flippant tone in the pages of *Dancing on Quicksand*, it is a result of my having stood toe-to-toe with the dragon and discovered it is often helpful to laugh in the face of the beast.

—M.M.

Contents

Acknowledgments

To Heather Brooke and Trey Spangenberg: My treasured children, who, throughout their early years, tutored me in preparation for my time with David. To the adult Heather, who believed in me, wouldn't let me stop believing in myself, and taught me I always have options. How did you grow to be so wise, Darlin'? To the adult Trey, for his knowing glances, tender, calming energy, humor that leaves me gasping, and 'round-the-clock computer wizardry that keeps me cyber-nimble.

To Chris Russell: Long-devoted friend, listener, nettler, and encourager who envisioned this book and refused to hear my reluctance to write it.

To Kathy Bowers: Steadfast, can-do friend, flag waver, smart and fearless reader.

To Brian Cruce: Friend extraordinaire, whose indefatigable eye and ear for word and nuance allowed me to sound smarter than I am—the one I've called on too often and usually later than I should.

To Holly Brooks and John Sturtz: My cousin and her partner who courageously read and meticulously commented on the first draft, then stood by with support of every sort.

To Benjamin Thompson: My burst-of-light, visionary, philosophizing friend who witnessed moments with David that others only heard about.

To Cheryl Meyer and Daniel Lynch: The very first readers and tireless cheerleaders.

To Tina, Harrison, Desolina, and Cruz: My cherished family-next-door—my earth tethers.

To Adele Brodkin: Crafter of my custom-made Dumbo's feather.

To Sara Duncan: Erstwhile friend, current friend, and writing-seed planter.

To Wayne Ewing: A remarkable stranger who paused long enough to recognize our kindred spirit then directed me to Ellen.

To Ellen Kleiner: Who welcomed me warmly, straightened my collar, and sent me to Stephany.

To Stephany Evans: My agent and now beloved friend who "got it" when others didn't, then "ran with it" and ran, and ran, and … is still running.

To Mira Perrizo and Stephen Topping at Johnson Books: My publishing family who understood David's story, believed it had value for others, and resolved to publish a book uncharacteristic of their catalog. Mira won my heart with her serene presence, her patience with this first-time author, and her prowess as an eleventh-hour, tall-building leaper.

To David Morgan: New friend and insightful editor who encouraged me to blend more of my own experience into David's story.

To Other Early Readers: Maryanne Alexander, Sylvia Anholtz, Tara Bardeen, Marcia and Richard Baum, Adele Brodkin, Ruth Brunner, Annie and Daniel Cohen, Sandy Conheim, Douglas Cooper, Lois and Alan Fern, Bill Gold, Marion Gottesfeld, David and Shelly Hiller, Sara and Harvard Holmes, Terry Katz, Peter Lambert, Tom Lambert, Gladys and Bill Ligon, Cathy McCabe, Michael Neil, Jim and Lucia Rayburn, Keith Rich, Marijane Sharpe, John Simonet, Marion and Bill Smith, Ellen Steinberg, Pegi Touff, Liz Waggener, Ruth Wohlauer. Heartfelt thanks to all of you, and to the many other early readers I've never met, whose interest in David's story fueled my belief in my project.

And ultimately, to the Touff Family: Terry, Michael, Sissy, and David himself, who welcomed me into their family circle, entrusted me with David's adventure agenda, and eventually with a great deal more. They unflinchingly encouraged me in my efforts to tell David's story. I am ever and lovingly grateful.

Beginnings

OVER A SPAN OF EIGHT YEARS, a few of my patient friends listened to regular installments of "The David Adventures" and witnessed my personal evolution. They believed I was gaining insight that might hold inspiration or solace for others, and urged me to put David's story into writing. Having never written a book, I was initially reluctant to embark on such a project. Yet I warmed to the idea of writing David's story as I rationalized that throughout my life, I have not been "qualified" to do most of what I have undertaken—including rollicking through adventures with an elderly gentleman who was sliding into dementia. When I finally began to write, tears, laughter, and written words poured forth in cathartic torrents and I knew I was on to something—for myself if for no one else.

Emboldened by my first draft, I broke the rules of courtesy and friendship and asked my prodders to read what I had rendered—fair reprisal for their prodding. Their responses were swift and encouraging. Without my knowledge, they passed that first manuscript to spouses, children, and friends. Soon I was receiving requests for additional copies. Next, I was fielding calls from strangers across the country who wanted to express their appreciation for David's story, or to ask my opinion (*my* opinion?) about their own situations. By the time there were two hundred "David" manuscripts adrift in the land (all having issued from my beleaguered printer), I realized I was sharing my home, office, and time with a seemingly separate entity—The Book—that had its own agenda.

PERHAPS THERE WILL BE readers who want to see more of my own angst in the following pages—to witness more of my turmoil in order to measure the validity of my words. So I want it known that although I am generally a patient and optimistic person, my patience and optimism were constantly tested as David and I journeyed together, and whatever insights I gained were tempered by the harsh realities of ever-present and frustrating challenges. But if I had focused here on my own disquiet, *Dancing on Quicksand* would have become more my story and less David's. While David's is the more compelling story, I don't want to leave readers with the impression that I sailed through our adventures without a ruffled feather. To paint this picture would trivialize the daunting struggles of the multitudes of individuals— family members and professional caregivers alike—who daily labor at the formidable task of caring for those who have dementia. From the beginning of my association with David, I have been clear that my ruffled feathers did not belong on his doorstep; I took them instead to my stalwart friends who unfailingly smoothed them.

I would be the first to acknowledge that in matters of caregiving, my perspective is limited, because I am neither a family member nor a full-time caregiver. And experience has convinced me that I am not cut from the steel cloth that is required of one who is devoted to full-time caregiving. I learned this during some of our more trying moments on the road and when David came to live with me for a month. Over the years, the thing that best enabled me to maintain my poise (on most occasions) was the knowledge that my hours with David, though regular, were limited to a few at a time. I needed the awareness that the end was always in sight.

If *Dancing on Quicksand* makes any contribution, this one truth may be the most valuable nugget in the whole of David's story: Without respite, single-handedly caring for one who is affected by dementia is a perilous undertaking, and because this is so, caretakers must guiltlessly allow themselves to seek help.

David's wife, Terry, sought help. It was Terry who facilitated David's and my relationship over the years and Terry who gained my respect as she unfalteringly demonstrated her natural optimism, discipline, and extraordinary ability to carry on.

Some readers may question Terry's limited role in the pages of *Dancing on Quicksand.* I can say only that her lack of prominence is not a reflection of her relationship with David, but more a function of how the three of us structured our lives to best support both David and Terry. Although Terry was the one who initiated and welcomed my association with David, she was very much in the background of David's and my relationship. Often I would not even see her when I arrived to take David out. As David's dementia worsened, my relationship with Terry deepened, but my primary focus was still on David and relieving Terry of his constant care.

Terry is an energetic woman of action. She spends little time brooding and analyzing and rarely draws others into her inner tumult—nor does she dwell on it herself. Outsiders might interpret Terry's demeanor as detached or uncaring, but they would be mistaken. Terry is unwavering in her devotion to David, and David's constant references to her as he and I adventured together are testimony to their enduring bond. When I met the Touffs, they had been married fifty-nine years and their relationship was a billowing canopy that sheltered their graceful dance with each other—a loving and affectionate, respectful yet independent tango.

For every hour I spent with David, Terry spent many times that number of hours attending to David's every need, coping physically and emotionally with his decline. Within those hours surely lies another story, but that story would be Terry's to tell.

IN AN ARTICLE that appeared in *Creative Nonfiction,* Vol. 16, 2001, entitled "The Line Between Fact and Fiction," Roy Peter Clark states, "Scholars have demonstrated the essential fictive nature of all memory. The way we remember things is not necessarily the way they were. This makes memoir, by definition, a problematic form in which reality and imagination blur."

Dancing on Quicksand is something of a memoir and subject to the healthy skepticism voiced by Clark. Therefore, I want my readers to understand that I did not record conversations with David. I did not even keep a formal journal. Occasionally, I jotted down those things that stood out as unusual or special, but dialogues with David are reconstructed from my memory. Many of the dialogues are verbatim—I am enthralled by words and tend to remember them. But surely, over the course of eight years, I have not remembered every word accurately or in its proper sequence. However, I believe that throughout *Dancing on Quicksand* the dialogue between David and me is 100 percent true to personality, character, and circumstance.

As I wrote, it was my constant intention to maintain accuracy in content and chronology so the reader might chart the progress of David's journey. The progression may not always be apparent, since David's dementia has not followed a linear path. Yet it is, in part, the mercurial nature of his awareness and inconsistent behavior that has magnetized me and kept me steadfast in my resolve to be a supportive witness to his latter years. My watchfulness has always been abundantly rewarded with signals from David that his core remains intact.

David's niece, Lois Fern, after reading *Dancing on Quicksand*, wrote to me, "You have captured David to perfection. Not, of course, the brilliant, knowledgeable uncle I remember, but the shadow that retains the outline of the man he'd once been ... the degree to which he's held on to his essential personality. His values, his decency, his curiosity, and his humor have somehow remained intact, even though his memory has failed him."

That I never knew "the man he'd once been" yet "captured David to perfection" seems to validate the notion that his essence was present and that I have mirrored rather than invented that essence.

The format of *Dancing on Quicksand*, like our relationship, was shaped by David's dementia. The snapshot quality of the book's chapters is a microcosm of our years together and perhaps reflects the nature of dementia itself. To fashion a cohesive story from significant but disjointed fragments was a challenge. But what became clear to me early in my association with David was the importance and emotional richness of moments rather than how the moments themselves flowed together.

The Touff family graciously offered me the use of their names. David's doctor, Abe Kauvar; my friends, Kath and Chris; Linda, the waitress at the Fourth Story; and Amy, the librarian, are also authentically identified. I've created pseudonyms for all other characters in the book to protect their privacy. Also, for reasons of privacy, I created the name Willowglen for David's residence. Similarly, the names of all residents and staff at Willowglen are invented.

It seems that Alzheimer's disease has become the generic term for all types of dementia. But Alzheimer's is only one form of dementia—not all dementia is Alzheimer's. Certain tests and close observation of a patient's symptoms over an extended period of time can rule out Alzheimer's, but to date, only brain biopsy or autopsy can provide a definitive diagnosis. Therefore, throughout this book, I use the broader term, *dementia*, rather than *Alzheimer's*.

NO DREARY TALE OF bedpans and shrouded windows, *Dancing on Quicksand* is a story of respect, trust, and truth. Although dementia is the vehicle that brought David and me together, and in many ways defined the parameters of our relationship, adventure was the focus and driving force of our unusual union.

What follows is an account of one man's journey into dementia, a relationship that evolved as a result of that journey, and the surprising lessons the journey itself taught. David, by example, challenges all of us to participate more fully in our own lives; the bond we formed is a reminder of the sustaining nature and powerful, transforming potential of authentic human relationship.

Marilyn Mitchell
Denver, Colorado
2002

1

Square One

As You Wish

After twenty-five years of marriage, I am abruptly single and in a precarious financial position. My daughter is a freshman in college, I am rearing my eleven-year-old son, and I feel an urgency to devise a plan for my financial future. With no work history or credentials other than a quarter century of homemaking and mothering, community service, several marginally successful entrepreneurial ventures, and the patent to a gardening implement I've invented, I don't qualify for the jobs that will pay me what I need to meet my expenses.

But I'm forty-six years old and have mastered many life skills, so I create As You Wish, a personal service business—a vehicle for offering my particular talents to a select clientele. My brochure lists services as diverse as "landscaping, checking on grandma, decorating your home for the holidays, writing your most difficult letter, chauffeuring your kids to soccer practice, taking bids for your new roof, or finding a belly dancer for your party."

One scorching July day, while landscaping a Denver street corner with a crew of laborers, I notice an attractive, vigorous-looking couple in their eighties getting out of a car across the street. The woman, a silver-haired, brown-eyed pixie, casual but chic in jeans, approaches me with a barrage of friendly questions and introduces herself as Terry Touff. Soon satisfied with my answers, she takes one of my brochures, briskly rejoins her husband, and they hurry off to a matinee at a nearby theater.

The following April, Terry calls and reintroduces herself. She explains that for the past thirty years, during the month of May, she has worked three days a week at a local greenhouse. She wants to continue her springtime tradition, but is concerned about leaving her husband, David, alone. David, eighty-nine years old, is accustomed to being active, but he has recently stopped driving. With Terry at work, he will be stranded at home with no diversions.

Terry's question: "During the month of May, will As You Wish create and facilitate three adventures a week for David?"

My answer: a casual "Yes," but my mind is racing: *A guaranteed month of work—a small net of safety. Thank you, Terry Touff, whoever you are.*

That May turns into years. As mutual trust and respect grow, Terry delegates more responsibility for David's care to me. She herself is aging and unable to single-handedly give David the support he needs. She also wants to minimize the burden of David on their two children who have families and careers to attend to.

When I agree to Terry's proposal, I do not know that David is in the early stages of dementia—perhaps Alzheimer's. David's diagnosis is so recent that neither he nor Terry has had time to fully accept the harsh reality of their situation. So I do not suspect that soon the three of us will be catapulted into mental and emotional quicksand as our lives converge, then perpetually shift; that a relationship with David Touff will teach me vital life lessons and expand my ability to dance through adversity; and that adventures with David will provide an opportunity for me to test my limits and discover that my limits are far less confining than I had imagined.

David

In his prime, David was not a large man—only five-foot-six. At his current, shrunken height of five-foot-three, he is charmingly elfin in stature. The years have molded his posture into an asymmetry that lends a jaunty air to his demeanor. Unlike many men his size, David exudes a quiet self-confidence and gracious ease with the world. His eyes are that rare, intense blue that makes strangers look twice to confirm the reality of such blueness. The blush of good health colors his cheeks. When David smiles, he smiles with his whole face, and his radiant goodwill often magnetizes bystanders. David's hair is gray and well cut, his clothes vintage Brooks Brothers, his manner gregarious yet never imposing. Above all, David is genteel but entirely without pretense.

First Adventure

When I arrive at his house on the morning of our first adventure, David greets me cordially, but with obvious eagerness to set out. We are going to visit the Denver Museum of Nature and Science.

At the museum, David is immediately captivated by the dioramas and tireless in his quest to "see it all." He comments and questions with intelligent insight. But repeatedly David refers to his wife, Terry, saying, "I must bring Terry back here," or "Terry has no *idea* this tremendous place exists," and "Remind me to get a card from this place, so I'll be able to tell Terry where it is."

I'm thinking: *This doesn't make sense. We used David and Terry's membership pass today, yet David indicates this museum will be a revelation to Terry.*

Having met David only briefly prior to this day, I am not aware that he is in the early stages of dementia. Further, I do not know that, unrelated to his dementia, David has hand tremors that are severe enough to make his eating difficult and often embarrassing for him.

We go to the museum cafeteria for lunch. Before I am even seated, David spills his coffee, drenching himself and the table. Grabbing handfuls of napkins, I dam the deluge. Eventually equanimity, if not dryness, is restored. I bring David fresh coffee and a straw so he won't have to lift his cup off the table to drink. He pronounces me a genius. I've eliminated the whims of a palsied hand. If I had invented and manufactured straws on the spot, David could not be more in awe or more grateful. He acts as if he has never seen a straw.

Moments later the catsup bottle, wielded by David, takes an unexpected glug. He stares aghast at his shaking hand holding the bottle that is flooding his hamburger and fries. David's reflexes are sluggish, and he seems disoriented—frozen in this elongated moment.

"Just one of the mysteries of the universe, David—some catsup bottles are spring-loaded. I've had this same thing happen myself," I commiserate, retrieving his lunch from the thick red bog and transferring the salvage to a clean plate.

As we eat, I make small talk, referring to exhibits that particularly interested David in the museum. Oddly, the things that seemed to fascinate him only minutes ago are now inconsequential. What I have observed over the last several hours is troubling. I believe David has significant problems, although I don't understand exactly what they are.

Back home, our first priority is to walk Lovie, the Touffs' feeble, sixteen-year-old cockapoo. I notice that David cares for Lovie, but he's inept at handling her, insensitive to her needs. Lovie, blind and deaf, is even more frail than David. She is asleep on her cushion when he wrestles her up, stuffs her awkwardly under one arm, makes his way precariously down a long flight of stairs, moves haltingly out the front door and down the sidewalk to a grassy area. Abruptly, without bending down, he pitches Lovie unceremoniously to the ground. I'm stupefied. Have I just witnessed business as usual or is something out of the ordinary happening here? Doesn't this bizarre and laborious undertaking put both David and Lovie at risk?

Terry has asked me to stay with David just long enough for him to take care of the dog, but I am uncomfortable leaving David alone until Terry returns. I don't know if his behavior today is typical; perhaps he has suffered a mild stroke. Terry may be unaware of his condition. I have too many unanswered questions. My dilemma is further complicated, because my next client, a woman I've never worked for, will be expecting me soon. But I decide that leaving David would be irresponsible. I call the woman, tell her something has come up, and I'll be delayed.

David overhears my call and says good-naturedly, "Go on now. I don't need a babysitter, for God's sake!"

I stall, pick up a magazine, and comment with interest on an article about Native American weaving. David becomes interested too, or maybe he is just being a gracious host.

Shortly before Terry is due to return, I put on my coat to leave. David ushers me to the door, thanks me with genuine gratitude for "our wonderful day together," and tells me conspiratorially, "I think you're gorgeous, but you don't need to worry; I'm too old to get either one of us in trouble."

Cute, but what have I signed up for? Before our next escapade, I need to learn much more about David.

LATER, I CALL TERRY. She acknowledges that David has certain challenges. I sense that she does not realize, or has not fully accepted, the scope of David's impairment. Terry insists that David is capable of staying alone after I leave him. I feel uneasy with this arrangement. But Terry has lived with David longer than I have *lived*. Who am I to tell her about his deficits? At least I have expressed my concerns. With this much definition I can continue.

Denver International Airport

David and I are off on our second adventure, this one a visit to the newly opened Denver International Airport (DIA). DIA is a novelty, and many people travel miles onto the prairie to "see the new airport."

Despite the gaps in his memory, David is exceptional in his curiosity and perceptiveness. Driving to DIA, he continuously comments and questions: the traffic, the condition of the highway, the industrial growth that sprawls along the I-70 corridor, the sort of companies that make up the sprawl, the long-term impact of the sprawl, the distance from the heart of the city to the airport, the prairie vegetation, and on and on.

Arriving at DIA, we immediately agree that there is more to explore than we can cover in one visit. We begin in the main terminal.

The Jeppesen Museum captivates us for at least thirty minutes. There is nothing wrong with David's attention span when he is intrigued.

The main terminal is named after Elrey B. Jeppesen. Neither of us has heard of him. This alone sparks our interest. We learn that he was an aviation pioneer, famous for creating aviator maps that are still standard equipment in cockpits today. Jeppesen Sanderson, the company he founded, now grosses multimillions annually. Orville Wright signed Jeppesen's first pilot's license! Both of us could happily stay longer at this mini-museum, but there is much more we want to see.

From the lower level of the main terminal we can see three "sky bridges" bordered by a colorful balustrade. David has been eyeing this unique railing since we entered the terminal. We take the escalator to the upper level and discover that the balustrade is a magnificent, handmade work of ceramic art. For the remainder of our stay at DIA, David gestures toward the balustrade every time it comes into view. He says he'd "like to take a closer look," forgetting we've already studied it at close range.

We move on to a mural entitled *Children of the World Dream of Peace*. Long a serious collector of folk art, David is delighted by the detailed representation of folk costumes from around the world.

We ride the concourse train to the end of the line and back. David exclaims, "This technology is tremendous! Imagine having a high-speed, underground train to carry people to and from the airplanes! My God, I'm glad I lived long enough to see *this*!"

The throng, moving away from the train, carries us toward the escalator up to the main terminal. David gestures overhead and comments animatedly on the whimsy of the airplane mobiles that mark the way.

On the packed escalator David segues from flying mobiles to a loud and startling query: "If a fella had to do a bowel movement in a hurry, where would he go around here?" A voice from an unseen face answers, "Turn left and left again at the top." Then the entire airport falls silent.

A thought flashes: *Maybe I need to expand my brochure to include "willingness to endure extreme embarrassment."*

David emerges from the restroom beaming, exclaiming to all nearby and some beyond, "That is without a doubt the finest men's room I have ever used in a public place!"

He extols the cleanliness, the layout, the state-of-the-art fixtures. David's monologue is compelling. I'm sure there are men without previous inclination to visit the men's room who now hurriedly detour into that inner sanctum to see firsthand what this self-appointed barker is acclaiming.

I am eager to move along to lunch, but David sees a store that specializes in holographs. Childlike in his enthusiasm for the holographs, he says he wants to buy something for me. I demur and suggest that he buy something for Terry. He likes this idea. David buys two ballpoint pens—razzle-dazzle little souvenirs that have holographic designs on the cases. He presses one of them into my hand and begs, "Please, Dear, let me give you this." The pen is a $3 item, and I accept it so we can move on to lunch. David's desire and *need* to buy things for me will be a recurring and, at times, contentious issue between us.

At a self-serve café on the upper level of the terminal, we are choosing our sandwiches when I sense that David has a problem. Turning, I see that his face is scarlet, his mouth is slack and pouring drool, his eyes are fixed, unseeing. I position my face in David's line of vision. He looks eerily through me. His face is expressionless. I speak his name. He does not respond.

I turn for help to the cashier operating the concession. He shrugs helplessly and mutters something in a heavy foreign accent. Does he not understand what I am asking? Is he telling me that he can't leave the café to go for help? The area seems frighteningly deserted. I can't leave David. As I open my mouth to yell for help, a maintenance man approaches. I ask him to call for emergency assistance. Within moments, two paramedics arrive with a wheelchair.

We proceed to the airport infirmary. The medics do a preliminary evaluation. David's color returns to normal, and his eyes begin tracking. He attempts to speak—slurred, incoherent garble. Still, there is no indication that he recognizes me. The medics inform me that in circumstances like these, airport policy dictates that the patient must be taken by ambulance to a hospital. I know nothing about David's medical history or hospital preference. I send him to Rose Medical Center. It happens to be a good choice. All of his medical records are at Rose.

Driving to the hospital, I call Terry. She'll meet us at the emergency room.

At the hospital I find David on a gurney surrounded by medical personnel. He spots me in the crowd.

"I'll be damned! Hello, Dolly. Where did you come from? How did you know I was here? I helped build this place, you know. Does Terry know I'm here?"

A doctor enters with David's medical file and begins an examination. David comments incongruously, "That was a long time ago. No ... no ... no, not anymore, but it sure was at the time."

The doctor steps back, startled. Incredulous, he explains, "Out in the hall just now I read in David's file about the major abdominal surgery he had years ago. As I palpated David's abdomen, I silently, repeatedly asked the question in my mind, 'Is this tender? ... Is this tender? ... Is this tender?' I was so engrossed in my examination that it took me a moment to realize that David was answering the questions I had formed in my mind but had not spoken aloud."

All of us are hushed, mystified.

Exuberantly, David breaks the silence, "ESP. I guess I have ESP!"

Terry arrives. While she isn't overtly angry, it is obvious that she isn't pleased either. She greets David, tells him he looks fine, and asks him if he'll feel like going to the dinner party planned for that evening. "I don't know. I'm pretty tired right now," David chuckles.

Terry volunteers, "This is just a TIA. He has them sometimes. His doctor says they are nothing to worry about, certainly not anything that requires emergency room attention." (A TIA is a transient ischemic attack—a fleeting mini-stroke.)

Motioning me into the hall, Terry says, "This probably means you won't want to continue with David. Right?"

"Why not, Terry?" I ask.

"Well, I guess the TIAs just complicate things, make life uncertain."

"Life *is* uncertain, Terry. You or I could have a TIA as we stand here talking. Now that I know David has TIAs, I won't be so alarmed next time. We'll cope with them."

"I'm sorry I didn't tell you about the TIAs. David has them so infrequently, I didn't think to mention it."

This TIA is the harbinger of many more.

2

Beyond May

Expanding a Friendship

May ends, but I continue to spend time with David. As always, our purpose is adventure, and our adventures are varied.

THIRTY MILES SOUTH OF Denver, we trek around the Castle Rock Factory Shops. A retired retailer of ready-to-wear, David is fascinated by an entire mall of outlet stores. We see an IMAX movie. As far as I can tell, David sleeps through most of it, but when the lights come up, he declares, "That was a sensation!" A morning at the flea market is a great success. "My God, where do these people get all this crap?" is David's constant and loudly repeated question.

Garage sales are also a favorite. David enjoys seeing other people's discards, and he's a master at engaging our fellow shoppers in banter. We tour Coors Field, Denver's new major-league baseball stadium, where David has another TIA. We explore the newly renovated Denver Public Library; David is enchanted by the fossilized marble floors and approving of the contemporary western atmosphere. Hiking around the Denver Zoo to visit all the spring newborns is more exhausting than thrilling for him. We are at Brooks Brothers one day when David suggests to a woman shopper, "Try on that outfit. I bet it'll make you look thinner."

A trip to the Butterfly Pavilion and Insect Center is a disappointment. From the moment we enter, David wants to leave. His usual, intense curiosity is never piqued. He seems disoriented, and I suspect that he is affected by the warmth and high humidity in the observation areas.

Another day we lunch at the legendary Brown Palace Hotel, a national historic landmark and one of David's long-ago favorite watering holes. Standing in the center of the hushed, ornately elegant, nine-story-atrium lobby, David raises his trembling arms and sobbing, loudly wails, "My God, look at this place. I've always loved this place. What happened? Why don't I come here anymore? Where are all my friends?"

Gently, I usher David into one of the hotel's restaurants. Even before we are seated, the scene in the lobby is forgotten, and we enjoy an uneventful lunch.

One Indian-summer afternoon, we stroll along an esplanade that showcases a group of restored Victorian houses that lend their quaint charm and historic importance to the Auraria Campus. Auraria is a Denver metropolitan complex that accommodates two colleges and a university. David was a member of the original development group of Auraria. Although he does not fully comprehend his role in the preservation of the houses, David is pleased to hear that he played some part, and he appreciates the houses themselves. They serve as a link to his past and trigger animated reminiscences about his childhood in the small rural town of Freeland, Michigan, where his father owned the general store.

There are two small, filler adventures that never fail to produce raves from David. The drive-through car wash inspires the same comment every time: "Wow! This is terrific, amazing! I've never seen anything like this in all my life!" And the technologically mysterious drive-through ATM typically elicits, "My God, you're a genius. I could *never* do what you just did!"

At the Denver Art Museum, we make a game of finding all the pieces that have been donated in David's honor or that he and Terry together have donated: a few contemporary pieces and a number of pre-Columbian clay figures. One, a Colima dog, is David's favorite.

Each time we find another piece David whoops gleefully, "This is the best day of my life! Thank you, Dear, for bringing me here. We have to tell Terry about this!"

The first house David and Terry owned in Denver is another of our destinations. This once-small, white, frame house sits on a piece of real estate that is uniquely forested by a dense urban woods. Purchased by the Touffs in 1939 for $5,000 and immediately remodeled, the house still stands—an unpretentious tribute to their renowned good taste. Perennials planted by Terry sixty years ago still bloom and border the property. Curious to see if David has any recollection of the area, I say nothing as we approach the house. When the house is in full view, he says, "Hey wait a minute! I used to live here! Gee, it's great to be back! It's been a long time since I've been to Detroit!"

We continue on to Cranmer Park, the neighborhood park where the Touff children played as they grew up. I want David to see the drinking fountain the Touffs donated in memory of their late son, Danny, and to enjoy the Panoramic Overlook with its remarkable view of the distant Rocky Mountains.

In 1992 David and Terry financed the restoration of the overlook after vandals defaced this unique Denver landmark. The overlook is a semicircular, flagstone plateau, the outer sweep of which spans approximately 200 feet. Along the perimeter of the plateau's curve is a two-foot-wide, multicolored mosaic border. Within this border, every major peak that can be seen in the distance is represented not only by its name and elevation but also by its brass-outlined, miniature silhouette, inlaid in the mosaic. Plaques note the Touffs' contribution of the restoration funds and donation of the fountain. Reading the plaques, David jubilates, "Unbelievable! Fan*tastic*! Terry doesn't know about this! We *have* to bring her back here!"

Another day we visit the Denver Botanic Gardens. Our goal is to find a Frank Swanson sculpture, *Reflections II*, donated by David and Terry in 1985. Terry has told me it is displayed in a water lily pond.

When we finally locate the piece, I am surprised to discover that this large, travertine marble sculpture is one I have admired for years, yet never known its name. Looking at this simple, contemporary piece has always been something of a meditation for me. After only moments of focus, my mind invariably relaxes into mentally reuniting to wholeness the work's three component parts. Excitedly, I tell David how thrilled I am to learn of his association with this sculpture. All David can think of is telling Terry.

The Forney Transportation Museum is another "best day of my life" adventure for David. Seeing the antique cars tweaks his long-term memory and gives me a rare opportunity to experience a more competent side of David. He becomes my eloquent guide, recalling, as far back as his boyhood, the cars his family owned, and his own first car, an Overland, manufactured by Wrigley. David points out many features and subtleties I might have overlooked: the unique braying sound of early car horns, wide running boards seemingly designed for daring young riders, lush but impractical upholstery fabrics, and the almost exclusive use of the color black for early automobiles.

Not only does David enjoy seeing the antique vehicles, he is proud to be the articulate initiator of much of the afternoon's conversation. For a few hours he has a chance to remind himself of the other, brighter, more scintillating David—the David he felt so comfortable being for most of his life. (See Appendix A: Activities)

Looking Both Ways

Terry has joined some friends for lunch. David and I have spent the morning at the house. We've taken a walk, I've read a number of articles aloud from today's paper, and I'm almost finished trimming his nails.

"Well, David, it's 11:45. If I don't scramble into the kitchen and pull some lunch together for us, you're going to start looking for a new sidekick."

"God, I'm scared when I think about how much ground I've lost in the last six months. I hate to think how I'll look a year from now," David says, with no warning.

Stunned by this non sequitur, I hesitate before responding, "I'm glad you brought this up, David. I often wonder if you might want to talk about your situation."

David is silent, so I continue, "There is no doubt about the fact that you have lost ground, David, but what amazes *me* is that your personality hasn't changed since I first met you. You are still honest, generous, compassionate, curious, and ready for adventure. You appreciate beauty. You still have your wonderful sense of humor. You just can't remember what day it is or what you ate for breakfast."

David, now looking into his lap, is still silent.

"David, what is the scariest part for you, about your situation?" I ask.

There is a long pause before he answers, "Not knowing what to expect—thinking I might not recognize myself at some point."

"What you're describing sounds very scary, David. The truth is that none of us knows what to expect in this life. Every 'next moment' is unknown to all of us. But if our health is good and we have a little money in the bank, we aren't forced to look at our fears. Losing your memory is forcing you to look at how frightening the unknown really *is*. And by talking to me about your fear, you are being genuine. Many people go through their entire lives and never discover how to share their fears with another person. You've given me a precious gift, David. You have let me see that fragile part of yourself that not everybody gets to see. So even at this moment, in expressing your fear of losing yourself, you are living life more fully than a lot of people ever do."

"I guess you're right about that," David says, raising his head only slightly to look at me from under his brow.

"One thing you can count on in the days ahead, David, is that you will have love and support no matter what happens."

"Well, that's *something* to hold onto. Hey! What time is it? Is there a chance a guy could get something to eat around here?"

BECAUSE HE DOESN'T DWELL on his fears, I find it easy to forget that David has significant self-awareness and anxiety about his condition. I can imagine few terrors worse than knowing my mind is slipping away and not talking about it with those who are close to me. The mental deterioration itself would be overwhelming, terrifying. Not talking about my terror with people close to me would be isolating to the point of unbearable. I would need ongoing reassurance that I would be cared for and supported through my oblivion.

Today, David has drawn me in with his candor. Now that he's hooked me, I hope Terry will want me to be present as David continues his hard journey.

International Bell Museum

Soon after this conversation, we drive to the mountain town of Evergreen and, with difficulty, find the obscure little International Bell Museum in a 1919 historic house on a narrow, rutted road beyond Evergreen Lake. Unable to find any information about the museum before venturing out, we are unaware that it is open by appointment exclusively and only during the summer months. Fortunately, Winston Jones, the owner and curator of the museum, is on the premises and welcomes us in for a tour.

For two thrilling hours, we have a private, guided tour of the world's largest collection of bells—more than 6,000 of them—dating from 1000 B.C. to the present and ranging in size from a quarter inch in diameter to one ton in weight. Periodically, David refers to his *own* bell collection. Unaware of his collection, I am silently skeptical.

Of all the bells, one in particular, an ancient, cast-bronze Chinese bell with elaborate relief detailing, draws David back again and again. "I have a bell just like that," he declares repeatedly.

At home several hours later, David leads me into the dining room to see his prominently displayed bell collection. The collection is a diverse and charming assortment of bells from around the world. I wonder how I've missed seeing it.

David is perturbed. "Where is that one bell? You know that big one?" he measures the air with his hands.

"I don't know, David. I've never seen it, but I'll help you look."

Our search is long, and David becomes frantic, childish in his help-less frenzy. We eventually find the bell in a shadowy niche outside the guest bathroom. It appears to be identical to the antique Chinese bell at the museum.

THE THINGS DAVID REMEMBERS often startle me, and I believe he remembers more than he is able to express. He remembered his bell collection, he remembered to look for the collection when we returned home, and he remembered the Chinese bell, even though it was not displayed with the collection.

From the beginning I had been ready to dismiss the idea that David had a bell collection, because I have observed his tendency to engage in what I term "springing." Springing occurs over a span of many hours—a periodic and fleeting reference that is triggered by something heard or experienced earlier in the day. David will hear one word, for example, "Bangladesh," on the morning news. He then earnestly uses the word "Bangladesh" throughout the day to spring from one idea to another.

"Will we be eating lunch in Bangladesh?" David asks shortly after hearing the word for the first time that day.

Hours later he will inquire, "Didn't I take that photograph in Bangladesh?"

Still later he will say, "That chair looks like it came from Bangladesh."

Close to bedtime he may want to know "How will we get home from Bangladesh?"

I made the assumption that talk of a bell collection and a missing bell was springing, stimulated by his experience at the bell museum.

TERRY CALLS ONE DAY, asking without preamble, "Is there any-thing in the house you especially like—a picture, a piece of furniture that you fancy? I want to put your name on something right now so you'll be sure to receive it after we're gone."

"Terry, please don't draw me into this. I feel awkward and embar-rassed having you even broach the subject. If I name something, I'll feel like a vulture!"

"So you'll deny me the pleasure of knowing you'll receive something of ours after we're gone? Come on, humor an old lady!"

"Oh, let me think. May I tell you later? Nothing comes to mind immediately."

"No, I'll wait while you think."

"Grrrrr, Terry!" A long pause. "Okay, one thing is special to me because of its connection to David—the cast-bronze, Chinese bell outside the guest bathroom."

I tell Terry the story of our search for the bell—how for me, the bell symbolizes David's remarkable determination and his tenacious will to hang on to the disintegrating remnants of his mind.

"Done!" she says.

That afternoon, I call Terry to say I'll be dropping something off for her around two o'clock. Waiting for me, Terry hears the overhead garage door opening. Bell in hand, she steps with theatrical flourish from the house into the garage.

"Take it right now!" she demands. "There is no reason for you not to have it now. It's not like it will leave a bare spot on the wall. Let me be happy today, knowing you have it."

The bell now enhances a shadowy niche outside *my* guest bathroom. A dozen times David has seen the bell in my home. Invariably, he comments, "Hey, that's spectacular! I have one just like it!" I always explain that he is my benefactor. David is delighted to know he has given me something so fine. He'll have the pleasure of discovering this fact over and over again.

I cherish the bell. It reminds me to maintain a humble respect for this precious person whose reality I can only imagine.

Why Truth?

Honesty is the virtue I value above all others, but I must admit that in my dealings with David, I have often been tempted to bend the truth for the sake of expediency or simply to maintain a pleasant atmosphere. However, having witnessed David's confusion, frustration and anxiety, I have become convinced that my adherence to the truth is imperative. Hinging on the truth are David's emotional well-being, my own serenity, and the health of our relationship—a health that includes his trust in me and my respect for him. Three separate incidents illustrate my approach to truthfulness with David.

I've Lived Longer Than Most Men Do

Terry is out for the day, David and I are alone at the house, and he has been cantankerous all morning. Finally I say, "David, I understand that you are frustrated, but my patience with your mean-spirited attitude is waning. Maybe you need a break from me. I for sure need a break from you."

"Please forgive me, Dear. I am an old man—about twenty years older than most men get to be. I'm paying a price for this by being uncomfortable and unpleasant. I'm miserable, and I'm making everyone around me miserable. I'm not worth a damn. Darling, my best advice to you is 'Don't ever live to be this goddamned old!' How does a guy get out of this anyway?"

David's self-aware apology transforms my attitude. I'm back in the game. "It's not time to 'get out of this,' David," I assure him. "We need to find something at this moment that makes us both glad we're still alive. I'm glad to be here with *you* at this moment, David, candidly sharing our feelings with each other. I'm also glad to be warm in your beautiful home, protected by thick, insulated walls from the harsh cold. I enjoy the luxury of the thermal-paned windows that keep the cold at bay, yet allow the sun's warmth to reach us. I'm also glad that we will soon go downstairs together, and you'll keep me company while I prepare a delicious lunch. Then we'll eat like royalty. How's that?"

Smiling, David responds, "You make it sound pretty good—better than it is really, but I'll go along with it."

If I Have to Use That Walker ...

Supporting David when we take walks together is increasingly difficult. He has fallen several times at home, so I have brought a walker for him. He uses it sporadically and grudgingly. This particular morning I am urging him to use the walker and come with me to see springtime gardens in the neighborhood.

"If I have to use that walker, I won't go for a walk. Everyone will think I'm an old man."

"You *are* an old man, David. And anyone who sees you with this walker will not think less of you. They will admire you for having enough gumption to be out walking at age ninety-one!"

"You know what I like about you, Darling?"

"What's that, David?"

"I can always count on you to tell me the truth. You sure don't try to charm me! How old am I anyway?"

"You're ninety-one now, David."

"That can't be right."

"Well, you were born in 1905, and this is 1996. Do the math yourself."

"Well, I'll be damned. I think I *am* ninety-one! People aren't supposed to live to be this old ... are they? How the hell do I get out of here?"

A Dinner Party

Eight of us, close friends and family, are gathered for a quiet dinner party in David's home. Predinner conversation drifts into a friendly political discussion.

Trying to participate, David interjects, "Yes, but who won?"

"Well, there is no official contest, David, just the typical, ongoing, political tug-of-war," I answer.

"No, I mean the baseball game," David covers.

"I don't think the Rockies are playing tonight," I say.

"Oh sure, that's right," says David, who has virtually no interest in baseball and certainly does not follow the Colorado Rockies' schedule.

Later in the conversation, David interrupts with "This discussion sounds like it's getting too serious. Would any of you like a tour of the house?" An awkward moment follows. All present are well acquainted with the house and the many wonderful pieces of art and memorabilia collected by David and Terry during their years of world travel.

"That's a tempting offer, David, but I think we are moments away from sitting down to dinner," one savvy guest replies.

"Oh yes, I guess I knew that!" David bluffs.

At the dinner table, David becomes anxious about "the check." He wants to be sure that he gets the check. I'm seated next to him and try discreetly to explain that this is his home, and there won't be a check. He looks at me skeptically.

"This isn't my house! This is a restaurant!" he argues.

"David, look behind you. Here's your bell collection. This is your house. You are entertaining guests at a dinner party in your own home."

There is a long pause before he says, "I guess that's right." Not two minutes pass before he calls to the caterer, "Please, be sure that I get the check."

I catch the caterer's eye and nod exaggeratedly. Quick on the uptake, she says, "Definitely, Mr. T. I'll be sure you get the check."

My Truth Guidelines

Two simple guidelines govern my truth-telling with David: (1) In public: when necessary, spare David and others the embarrassment of absolute truthfulness; (2) in private: patiently and lovingly tell David even the hardest truths. (See Appendix E: Dance Steps for Caregivers.)

When truth is my touchstone, I can relax and be genuine with David—not only in my answers to his questions, but also in my feelings of love and compassion for him. I don't exhaust myself by contriving or sugarcoating information for David, feeling guilty about doing this, then trying to remember what I told him on the off chance that *he* will remember. Sometimes he *does* remember.

In a situation such as the dinner party, the guests at the table are uncomfortable and embarrassed for David. If, after prolonged agonizing on the subject, he actually arrives at solid comprehension, he will be profoundly embarrassed in front of his guests. I see no point in hammering away at the truth. So I support the lie that the caterer will give him the check.

In contrast, when I tell David how I feel about his irritable behavior, we are alone. For the health of our relationship, I believe it is important that we truthfully express our feelings. Although I initiate the exchange, I am astonished by David's level of candor and the insight he shares with me in response to my saying I need a break from him.

Again, when David objects to using his walker, we are alone. What a sham it would be for me to placate him with something like "If anybody sees you, David, they'll probably think that you have sprained your ankle and the walker is temporary."

Another area of truthfulness I practice with David is not pretending to understand him when I don't. Sometimes I am so uncertain of what David is trying to say that it is impossible for me to respond. When this happens, I don't ignore him, and I don't fake it. I simply say, "I'll have to ask you to repeat that, David. I'm confused."

Invariably, David laughs and responds, "That makes two of us. At least half the time *I* don't know what the hell I'm talking about!"

Taking this honest approach with David conserves my energy. It lets him save face when he is lost in his mental maze. And it ends in laughter—laughter at humor David himself creates!

If I were in the throes of dementia, I imagine that I would want to have a sense that people were being truthful with me, that they were not discounting or patronizing me. Therefore, I try to be a constant, grounding influence for David, reflecting to him as much reality as I am able. I am never afraid that I will upset him by giving him too much truth, and I have told him some of the hardest truths of his life, over and over and over.

Frequently, I have observed others attempting to skirt the truth with David. Not only do I witness a rise in his anxiety level at these times, but I also see that those who are not being truthful are also unmistakably condescending toward David. These people underestimate him. David's memory has failed, but he remains keenly perceptive. The condescension (most evident in tone of voice and frozen, saccharine expression) is always a tip-off for David that someone is trying to hide something from him. Sometimes what people are trying to hide is nothing more than their own discomfort at being in his confused presence. I am convinced that David senses truth and is relieved when people confirm it for him.

Yet there are moments when I question my dedication to the truth. Lacking memory, David forgets a reality before he has time to adjust to it. For example, he cannot remember that his parents have died. Each time he questions me about them, I truthfully tell him that they are no longer living. Essentially, I am breaking the news of their deaths to him for the first time. Repeatedly subjecting him to this emotional dagger feels so harsh. Would it not be kinder to simply slide over the subject and spare David this painful reality? Sometimes he cries, sometimes he is angry because no one has told him, other times he is disbelieving and argumentative. In all cases, I tell him I wish I could offer gentler, more comforting answers to his questions about his parents. Then I remind him that he and I have always told each other the truth, and truth has made our friendship strong. Without fail, David responds with solemn gratitude and confirms that he wants only the truth from me.

Given his keen intuition, I am convinced that if I told David anything less than the truth, he would sense my deceptiveness. Then the bond that has taken us years to cement, and serves us so well, would surely begin to crumble.

One especially difficult aspect of my years with David has been spending time with him in the presence of his friends and family. As others try to shield him from the truth, I observe his heightened anxiety. I must constantly choose among remaining silent, contradicting these people (this further confuses David), and finding ways of expressing myself that don't compromise my philosophy of truth-telling. Guarding my every word in the presence of others exhausts me.

Further, since people are often uncomfortable in David's presence and few are committed to interacting with him beyond the superficial pleasantries, he is soon left to frantically tread and flail in swiftly moving social waters. It is natural for me to engage with others, but my being distracted leaves David unsupported. Watching his confusion, anxiety, and embarrassment is painful for me. After a three-hour social gathering, I feel more depleted than I do after spending a full day alone with David.

Telling David the truth doesn't ensure that he will feel no pain or anger. In fact, it guarantees that he will feel a broad spectrum of emotions. To this end, David does his share of crying and raging. My charter is not to deny him his emotional life but to support him in the fullness of his life, emotions and all.

David's mind has lost the boundaries of memory, the boundaries each of us relies on to anchor us securely to our lives. His loss must be accompanied at times by inexpressible terror—a mental free fall. He has no sure way to verify his own truth. There are moments when I suspect he wonders if anyone can be trusted to venture with him into the tormenting dungeons of his own mind. It seems reasonable to me that David might occasionally express his terror as anger. I am surprised that he doesn't spend his days in a constant state of rage.

Because David doesn't have his own truth, truthfulness from others is imperative. Without truth, he has nothing solid to grab on to as he careens out of mental control. I view myself as a repository for as much of David's history and truth as he and his family have entrusted to me. As he drifts further and further from reality, he still trusts me to delve with him into his treasury of truth and memory.

Highland's Garden Café

There are several restaurants that David especially enjoys. One is the acclaimed Highland's Garden Café, where we are having lunch. Suddenly, David takes us into what I call a loop. This time it's the "Jewish loop." Although not an observant Jew, David has recently become obsessed with his Jewish heritage.

"How did you find this wonderful Jewish restaurant, Dear?" he asks as we peruse the menu.

"I forget how I first heard of this place. But it's not a Jewish restaurant, David."

"You're wrong there, but I'm not going to argue with you," he laughs. Then looking for someone to side with him, he calls to one of the staff, "Say, waiter, is this a Jewish restaurant?"

"No, sir," the startled young man answers.

"Well, how many Jewish people are eating here right now?"

"I have no idea, sir," the waiter answers, hustling in our direction, no doubt hoping to lower the volume of the query.

"You could count them," David suggests, chuckling but only half teasing.

"David," I intervene, "you are asking the impossible from a busy man."

"Thank you, sir," I say, smiling at the waiter, and a flicker of understanding passes between us.

Our food arrives.

"Wow! Look at this. Great presentation! What a knockout!" David exclaims.

Then reengaging the same hapless waiter, he asks, "Is all of this kosher?"

"Uh … I'm not sure, sir," the waiter answers uneasily.

"Well, this is a Jewish restaurant!"

"Not really, sir."

"Well, I think you're wrong there."

"Thank you. We're keeping you from your other guests," I say, rescuing the waiter for the second time.

While we eat, David persists, "It's amazing, you'd never know by looking that all these people are Jewish."

"They aren't all Jewish, David, but does it matter one way or another?" I ask.

"I suppose not," he concedes.

After lunch, on the sidewalk outside the restaurant, we approach two women with toddlers in strollers. Leaning down to one child, David effuses, "What a beautiful little Jewish girl! I hope you're hungry, because you're in for a treat." Pointing toward the restaurant, he informs, "Best Jewish food I've ever tasted!"

I attempt to enlighten the two confounded women with a sympathetic expression and a slight nod. Taking David's arm, I steer him away from other pedestrians. We move quickly toward the car. I try to put a ceiling on the number of people we bewilder in one day.

BEING WITH DAVID IS teaching me to separate myself from another person's identity. There are still times when I squirm, but I am realizing that I am not an extension of someone else. David is David; I am Marilyn. Most people can see that David is handicapped in some way. They probably view me as more "normal," but what if they don't? Not worrying what others think frees me to be more helpful to David—less distracted by constantly looking over my shoulder trying to gauge the disapproval of onlookers—less fearful that I will be disdained or ostracized by virtue of association with one who is often socially awkward or inappropriate. Increasingly, I can relax and give David the benefit of an unencumbered heart—one that is tender and open toward him.

The Fourth Story

David and I have been to The Fourth Story restaurant many times. Invariably he declares, "This is my favorite place to eat!" Perhaps what David finds so appealing is more than the creative cuisine—delicacies from carrot ginger soup to frangelico cheesecake; more than the restaurant's location on the top floor—the fourth story—of the renowned Tattered Cover Book Store in the posh Cherry Creek area of Denver. Knowing David, my guess is that what he most enjoys is basking in the vitality that swirls around the diverse and dynamic people he sees sharing animated conversation. Maybe lunching at the Fourth Story is a way for David to feel he is still a part of that mainstream energy.

Over the span of several decades, the Tattered Cover, one of the nation's largest independent bookstores, has become a Denver institution. Owned by the Tattered Cover, The Fourth Story takes its decor from the bookstore itself. Shelves of books and well-worn antiques surround diners who are free to browse, take books to their tables, and put them on their dining tab.

David seems relaxed, yet invigorated by the serene, quietly buzzing atmosphere as we make our way through the bookstore and up to the Fourth Story. Everywhere he looks, something captivates him: a particular title, an inviting old chair and reading lamp, and, of course, the sheer immensity of the inventory.

On a clear day the mountain panorama from The Fourth Story includes Pikes Peak, located seventy miles to the south. The Fourth Story staff knows us, and, whenever possible, they seat us by a window where David appreciates the view and the sunshine.

We have just been seated when David comments, "I am surprised that the faculty dining room isn't busier at this time of day."

"Oh, wow, David. Where are we?" I ask.

"Aren't we in the faculty dining room at the University of Michigan?"

"We are at The Fourth Story Restaurant in Denver, Colorado."

"Whaaaat?" he yowls, scowling at me.

"Yes, here's the name and address of the restaurant on the menu."

"Well, I'll be damned! How did we get here?"

"We live here in Denver—your house is three minutes from here."

"No! I live in Michigan."

"We both live in Denver, Colorado, David. You were born and grew up in Michigan. As a young man, you lived and worked in Detroit, but you moved to Denver in 1937."

"Wow!" he says, laughing, "you're telling me things I never knew about myself!"

Linda, one of our favorite servers, arrives to take care of us. "Hi, you two! Good to see you both. David, how are you doing?"

"Wait a minute! How do you know my name?"

"We've met before, but it's been awhile. I'm so glad to see you again."

"By the way, Dear, are you a student here at the university?" David asks Linda.

We talk about other things, but throughout our entire lunch, David reliably returns to the University of Michigan. He can't remember where we are, but he has no trouble remembering to return to his Michigan loop.

Lunch finished, we're ready to go. David wants to leave a generous tip. He *always* wants to leave a generous tip. Amazingly, he has a good sense of what "generous" means in current dollars. "Here," he says, proffering a $10 bill, "put this on the tray." Then he asks me, "Do you have one penny? I want to leave one penny with the $10. That'll make her happy."

Later, I learn that adding one penny to a tip for exceptional service is an old custom.

Looping

When David is looping, I do my best not to discount him in any way. In the course of one lunch, I may answer the same question two dozen times. Why should I care? I know the answer! And talking about anything at all gives David a sense of normalcy. We are two people having lunch in a lovely restaurant—exactly like the other people around us, conversing amiably.

Although I have been tempted, I don't join David in his fantasy. I would never say, "Yes, it *is* surprising, David. One would expect that the faculty dining room at a large university like this would be more crowded at the height of the lunch hour."

My sole purpose when I am with David is to focus on and support him. I bring myself to only this one moment. Without boredom, I am engrossed in the process. But my focus and resolve are bolstered, because I know that my time with David is well defined. In a few hours I will leave him.

Springing and looping, though both are manifestations of forgetfulness and confusion, are different from each other. When David is looping, his mind spins in tight, obsessive circles. When he is springing, he remembers for an entire day a single word or phrase that he has heard in passing. Periodically he threads this word or phrase into the conversation.

Looping and springing fascinate me, because they seem contradictory to each other—indicative of problems at opposite ends of the confusion spectrum. It is difficult for me to understand how looping and springing can be symptoms of the same mental affliction—how they can be contained within the same mind.

It seems more logical to me that David would remember the relevant, present moment rather than a random word he heard many hours earlier. However illogical it may seem, the fact is that David remembers for a whole day something of no apparent consequence, while increasingly he forgets the pertinent present.

As we drive away from a restaurant, our appetites sated, it is not unusual for David to ask, "When in the hell are we going to eat?" Sometimes he is testing my sense of humor—most of the time he isn't.

OFTEN I OBSERVE A good-humored nonchalance in David's looping behavior. Other times I see that his looping makes him anxious—pushes him to the verge of terror. These terrifying loops are usually about his family relationships or his geographic location. When I sense impending terror, I feel compelled to intervene.

The most effective way I have found to ease David out of a loop is to engage him in another subject. But when attempting to redirect his attention, I always alert David so that a non sequitur won't further confuse him.

"David, I'm going to change the subject. Do you remember your boyhood piano teacher, Miss Vincent?"

"My God! I haven't thought of her in years! She was a wonderful lady. Every Saturday I rode the train to Saginaw for my piano lesson."

"How long was the train ride?"

"Oh, about an hour each way. I think it was only a twelve-mile ride, but the train made so many stops."

"Did you mind giving up so much time every Saturday for a piano lesson?"

"No, not really. That's just the way it was. By the way, Dear, what time does our train leave for Saginaw?"

The peril of another loop threatens. I answer, "We're in Denver, David, but let's change the subject. Let's talk about the great apple pie they serve here. Apple pie is still your favorite, isn't it?"

"And how!"

"Would you enjoy a piece of hot apple pie before we drive into downtown Denver?"

"Sounds like a wonderful idea! And some decaf with it."

David's anxiousness is dispelled. The pie and coffee arrive.

To the server David exclaims, "Wow! That's gorgeous, but why are you bringing it to *me*? I didn't order pie … did I?"

THE MAGNETISM OF A LOOP is strong and continues to pull on David's mind while I try to tug it in a different direction. In an effort to calm his anxiety, there have been times when I have caught myself tugging so hard against David's loop that I feel I've created a loop of my own—the "obsessing to pull David out of his loop" loop!

When this happens, I say, "David, I'm going to stop talking for a few minutes and just enjoy this wonderful food (view, sunshine, music, or whatever else a circumstance offers for me to "enjoy"). I'm not enjoying it as much as I want to, because I'm too distracted by trying to keep up with our conversation."

David is accepting of my withdrawal, but of course he soon forgets why we are silent, and he begins again. Social by nature, he is intolerant of long silences.

California Café

We are eating lunch at the California Café, an upscale Denver eatery. I regret coming, because David is in the first stages of a cold. Normally under these circumstances, we would have stayed home. But Terry is entertaining a group of women for bridge and wants to have the house to herself. As we sit waiting for our food, David's cold seems to worsen. All of his pockets are stuffed with tissues. He sneezes convulsively, dabs incessantly at his nose, and puts his used tissues on the table.

"David, this is a lovely restaurant. Putting your soggy tissues on the table is unappetizing, inappropriate," I say quietly.

He ignores me.

"David, I just spoke to you; did you hear me?"

"Yes," he monotones.

"We need to figure out something else to do with your dirty tissues, David."

He does not respond.

"David, why don't we move all of your clean tissues into one pocket so we can put all of your dirty tissues into the other pocket?"

"For God's sake, I'm not going to put dirty tissues in my *pocket*," he growls, louder than I would like.

"David, putting dirty tissues on the *table* is *worse* than putting them in your pocket. Leaving your dirty tissues on the table is unfair to me and to all of the other guests around us. If you won't put your dirty tissues into your pocket, then at least move them to that empty chair beside you until our waiter can bring us a paper bag for the tissues."

David stares at me. Finally, he moves the tissues to the chair.

Our food comes, but David is so congested that he has difficulty eating. He chokes. He coughs. He gags. His tremor is worse than usual. He is spilling food and drink on himself and the tablecloth. I clean up the messes and try matter-of-factly to support him.

David puts down his fork. With tears glistening in his eyes he says, "You don't have any idea how humiliated I am to be in a place like this with a beautiful woman like you—to have you see me making such a mess of myself."

I'm taken aback by his flash of self-awareness. "I know it must be very painful for you, David, but we've seen a lot of hard times together. We'll get through this."

But lunch seems interminable. Thinking about my future with David and the prospect of many more days like this feels overwhelming. I remind myself that one day in David's life is just one day. Each day dawns new. I must not tighten my perimeters of hope for David by mistakenly assuming that new lows are permanent lows. Certainly I would not choose to be defined by *my* worst day!

GENERALLY, I use David's name more often than I would in everyday conversation with others. When we are facing any sort of challenge, such as the day at the California Café, I use his name even more frequently.

Having observed David over time and in a variety of circumstances, I know that in difficult moments, repeatedly using his name effectively grounds him in the present and reminds him, on some level, that he and I are connected. I am not a stranger, I know his name, and hearing his name anchors him.

Similarly, because David frequently has trouble remembering from one sentence to the next (or even from the beginning to the end of the same sentence) what we are talking about, I deliberately repeat the subject as we go along. So in talking about his dirty tissues, I repeat the words "dirty tissues," not only from sentence to sentence, but sometimes within the same sentence.

As cumbersome as this repetitious way of speaking sounds, it is very helpful for David. It slows the pace of the conversation, making it easier for him to follow. By continuously identifying what we are talking about, I help to eliminate the possibility of confusion.

The same principle applies to the use of pronouns. I try to limit the use of words such as *it, that, he, him, she, her, they, them,* because these words are abstractions, and do not identify the subject. If David has *forgotten* the subject, he is scrambling to find meaning. When he discovers that the subject has turned into they, she, or it, he tends to give up.

To an outsider, this pattern of speech sounds condescending, like dialogue from an old *Dick and Jane* book. For David, my habit of frequently repeating the subject significantly increases his ability to follow and participate in a conversation, because he has a way to keep track of what's being said.

COUNTLESS TIMES I have been impressed by David's startling moments of self-awareness against the backdrop of his seeming oblivion. Now, years after the fact, I make a connection between the California Café experience and our first adventure—the spilled coffee, the runaway catsup. That bit of misery was on the first day of our relationship, in the early days of David's decline. Having learned how sensitive he is, I know he must have felt acutely embarrassed by the scene at the museum. Mishaps are more humbling in front of strangers than with trusted friends. That long-ago day David was stoic; I mistook stoicism for lack of comprehension.

Give That Man a Dollar

Like other large cities, Denver has a homeless and indigent population. Regardless of our destination, we see members of this sad multitude inhabiting urban corners, their humbling stories condensed to one-liners scrawled on tattered cardboard. David is perpetually dismayed by this troubling sight. His typical response goes something like, "Oh no! Look at that poor guy. He needs help. Quick, hand him some money."

Nearly childlike in his innocence, David sees only the immediacy of another human being in distress and feels compelled to help. We have many philosophical discussions about this wrenching problem—the fact that some of these people are mentally ill, many are substance abusers, and others are just scammers. We talk about how our money won't feed, clothe, or shelter those who are addicted; it will simply support their addictions. We also agree that mental instability, addictions, or whatever reduces people to begging on street corners doesn't make them undeserving of our compassion—that their problems are not only enormous for them individually but also for the society that harbors them.

In the end, I am always the curmudgeon who resists handing out the money. Instead I offer flat, intellectual words like "David, this is a social problem that won't be solved by dollars doled out to every needy person we see."

But as we sit at red lights, I avert my eyes from the eyes of the beseechers just outside my car door and wait uneasily for green lights to flash us on our way to beautifully appointed, air-conditioned restaurants where delectable food awaits us.

It is a blistering summer day when we see a man holding a sign that reads, "Let's face it, I need a beer."

Jubilantly, David hoots, "Hey! There's an honest man! Give him a dollar!"

I do.

A Promise

Out for a walk one morning, our conversation has been the usual disjointed, looping, mental meandering. Abruptly David stops, turns, and looks directly into my eyes. Tremulously, he grips my arm.

Tears well in his eyes, and his voice quavers in fervent tones, "Promise me that when I'm gone, you'll take care of Terry *exactly* the same way you've taken care of me. She's going to need you. Gee, I love that little girl! Will you promise me?"

3

Terry Is Away

Five Days on Our Own

Although Terry is eighty-four years old, she has always been fit, attractive, vibrant, and exceptional in her outlook and energy. Tennis, walking, gardening, the theater, entertaining, and traveling have always been a part of her normal routine. Being responsible for David has deprived her of her vital lifestyle. Eagerly she seizes the opportunity to participate in a five-day architectural tour of Chicago.

Terry has just left for the airport. David is agitated and sulking.

"You're acting like an irascible old man, David," I chide. "The way you're treating me, I think you're forgetting that we're on the same team."

"Oh, hell, I'm not mad at you, Dear. I'm mad at my wife. What's her name?"

"Her name is Terry."

"Terry? Well, Terry has no business leaving me. She belongs here. Not going on an airplane flying off to God-knows-where, away from me, damn it! And having you stay with me—this makes me feel like a baby."

"I can understand why you feel this way, David, but the upside is that with me here, you don't have to cook for yourself!"

"I'm not hungry anyway."

"That makes sense. You just finished breakfast."

"Breakfast? What time is it?"

"It's 9 A.M."

"At night?"

"No, nine o'clock in the morning."

"That can't be. It's nighttime."

"Look outside, David."

"Yes, so?"

"Well, the sun is shining."

"Yes, what about it?"

"It's daytime, not nighttime."

"I don't know what the hell you're talking about. I'm going upstairs to read my *Wall Street Journal*."

Bedtime

"Am I going to stay alone tonight?"

"No, David, I would never leave you alone."

"Well, you can't stay with me, in my house, at night! I don't know about you, but I have my reputation to consider! What will people *think*?"

"Everyone who knows will be glad that you have a good friend to keep you company while Terry is out of town for a few days."

"Where will you sleep?"

"I'll sleep in the bedroom down the hall."

"Will you leave the door open?"

"Do you want me to leave the door open?"

"Of course, I might need your help! You won't hear me if the door is closed."

"Then it's settled. I'll leave the door open. If you need my help in the night, call me. I'll hear you and come running. You probably don't know this, David, but my sprint is unrivaled this side of the Mississippi."

"That's good to know," he chuckles.

"Good night then, David. Sleep well."

"Wait a minute! 'Good night?' Just like that? You're not coming in after I'm in bed to say a proper good night, maybe even give me a kiss?"

"I'd *like* to say a proper good night, David. Call me when you're ready."

Soon, he calls. I sit on his bed for a few minutes. We talk about tomorrow's forecast, the night-light that helps him find his way to the bathroom in the dark, whether he has enough blankets. I give him a kiss and a long hug, walk to the bedroom door, and turn out the light.

"Thank you, thank you, thank you, Darling. God, what would I do without you?"

"You're welcome, David. I'm glad to be here with you, and I appreciate being appreciated."

I go to my room and flop on the bed—limp, exhausted. As much as I've grown to love David, he challenges me, pushes me at times to the very edge of my patience and endurance. I am stressed, because I feel I must always be "on," vigilant: continuously trying to see things through his eyes, to anticipate difficulties before they arise, to avoid conflict without being condescending, to demonstrate my respect for David as a grown man, while needing, for practical reasons, to be aware that he has many childlike tendencies.

I lie on the bed looking at the ceiling. I've brought a book to read, but I lack the energy to get up and walk the short distance to my suitcase to unpack it. I continue lying motionless on the bed, letting the low ebb of my mental, physical, and emotional energies and the weight of the heavy, silent aloneness envelope me.

When the phone rings, I realize I've been lying in the same spot for forty-five minutes. At first, I don't recognize the shallow, almost inaudible, but labored voice of the caller. Straining to hear, I make out my sixteen-year-old son Trey's pleading, "Mom ... help. So sick ... please ... come."

My churning gut and pounding heart vie for attention. "Oh, Baby, I'm on my way. Be there in five minutes." The phone clicks off at Trey's end.

Trey had a slight sore throat this morning, but I wasn't too concerned. Now, sixteen hours later, he is seriously ill and needs my help, yet how can I leave David? I could call David's son, Michael, but it's late, and I'm embarrassed to disturb him with my personal problems.

God, help me. This is intolerable. I'm trapped. Caught up in an emotional avalanche, I'm only vaguely aware of the pain around my head, then realize I'm pulling my hair with both hands.

What shall I do? Quickly, I reason that Terry frequently leaves David alone. Maybe I can leave him briefly since he's asleep. I hurry to his bedroom door and listen to his even, deep breathing. I convince myself that he won't awaken while I'm gone. *Sleep, David.*

I run downstairs, throw on my coat, and tear out the door. I speed the mile to my house and leap the front steps by twos. *Sleep, David.*

I find Trey on the floor of his bedroom curled in front of a space heater. He is in his down sleeping bag, has pulled the quilt from his bed to pile on top of that, yet he's trembling with chills. I reach out to lay my hand on his forehead. Before I touch him, still several inches away, I can feel the heat radiating from his whole head. I take his temperature—103. His head is congested, his chest tight.

I ply him with cold juice and aspirin, set up the humidifier, and leave to go to the store for supplies. *Sleep, David.*

I return with juice, a decongestant, and Kleenex. I give him a dose of decongestant, pack a picnic cooler with ice, juice, and clean glasses, and put it within Trey's reach. Then I lie on the floor beside him, hold him, and for ten minutes we cry together. *Sleep, David.*

Trey has the cordless phone in his sleeping bag. I can think of nothing more to do for him, but *want* to do so much more—most of all I want not to leave him. *Sleep, David.*

"Oh, Sweetheart, it crushes my heart to leave you. Please call me if you need comfort. I can stay on the phone with you all night if that will help. I'll call you as soon as I'm back at David's."

"Mom … thanks … love you … oh … Mom … bye."

I walk toward the door. Turning to say a final good-bye, I see the mound of bedding heaving with Trey's silent sobs.

Driving back to David, I'm crying, raging, furious … at no one. It's painful enough to see Trey suffering. Being unable to properly care for and comfort him is agony.

Mercifully, David is still sleeping. I sleep a troubled sleep that is too soon interrupted by David's cheerful, early-morning greeting, "Well, *hel*-lo. What are you doing here?"

Over the next forty-eight hours, I bounce between Trey and David, feeling constantly like a thief for stealing time from either of them. But Trey quickly improves, and David and I soon take to the road.

Danny's Memorial

Over the years, it seems by osmosis, I have gradually learned a great deal of the Touff family history as well as David's singular history: his education, the path of his career, his community involvement, his travels, his passions. So I know that David and Terry had a son, Danny, who died in 1963, at the age of twenty-two, in a mountain-climbing accident.

One day, we drive thirty-five miles to the Boulder campus of the University of Colorado. Our mission is to find the garden and memorial sculpture the Touffs donated to CU in Danny's memory. At the time of his death, Danny was a chemistry student at CU. The sculpture is located in the courtyard adjoining the chemistry department. I have seen the eighteen-inch-tall maquette of this sculpture in the Touff's home, so I have some idea of what we are looking for.

We try to move in the direction of the chemistry department, but it is difficult to determine exactly which direction this is. Most people we ask say immediately that they can't direct us. Others believe they can, but they actually can't. The campus is large. At best, we must walk a considerable distance. Add in the backtracking we do, and our foray becomes an endurance test.

Trekking along, I marvel at David's enthusiasm and tenacity. Not only is the hike a challenge for him, but he has no vision of what we're doing, though I have told him several times.

Eventually we find the garden and monument. I explain repeatedly before David grasps the significance of what we are looking at. When he finally understands, he is overcome by emotion.

The bronze sculpture, a fifteen-foot abstract of a human figure with upraised arms, is installed in an elevated garden surrounded by a flagstone retaining wall. David wants to climb this wall to gain access to the sculpture itself. He is frenetic in his effort to reach the statue. I persuade him to give up his climb, go up the adjoining stairs, and enter the garden from the rear. Once in the garden, he strokes the statue and cries.

We spend probably ten minutes in this way. David speaks with intense emotion about Danny, expressing how grateful he is to be here paying tribute, how much he misses Danny, how sad he is even after so many years.

We try to read the inscription on the plaque. Years of weathering have tarnished it, making it difficult to read. David is distressed that no one has maintained the plaque. (When Terry returns from her trip, I tell her about our visit to the memorial and the deteriorating plaque. Immediately she arranges for the plaque's replacement.)

David takes an old day planner from his breast pocket. He attempts to write something in the front cover of the book, but his shaking hand makes writing difficult, illegible. Handing the book to me, he says, "Here, Darling, write it for me. Print it, will you? I want to be able to read it every day."

I print the simple inscription and read it aloud:

FLOWER ON THE MOUNTAIN
IN MEMORY OF
DANIEL LOUIS TOUFF
1941—1963

All the way back to Denver, David talks about Danny, the statue, and the inscription we wrote in his book. For the next two days our trip to Boulder and its significance are the predominant theme. Incessantly, David reads aloud the copied inscription in his book.

By the end of the second day, David is struggling to remember this important event in his recent past.

"Didn't we go somewhere?" he asks. "I think there's something important in my book," he says, producing his day planner. But he can't identify my printed entry as the important thing. Even with my assistance, David can't re-create what he longs for—as if watching the fading glitter after a burst of fireworks, he is helpless to recapture the glory of the previous moment. By the third morning after our trip to the memorial, he has no recollection of it. But even two days of retention is remarkable for David!

I SPECULATE THAT adrenaline plays a part in David's rare flashes of perception and his memory of some recent events but not others. I suspect that an adrenaline surge gives him a momentarily sharpened focus—a short-lived clarity. If the adrenaline infusion is of extended duration, it may also serve to imprint the brain and aid in extending the length of time an event is remembered.

Adrenaline is the universally recognized chemical trigger for the "fight or flight" mechanism. It is the chemical boost that facilitated the split-second reasoning required by our ancestors when deciding whether to fight the beast or flee from it.

Countless times, I have observed David as he emerges from confusion into clarity. Frequently, clarity occurs at times of physical or emotional excitement. I believe unusual stimulation activates an adrenaline response that impacts significantly and positively on his memory retention. While there have been moments of clarity without the observable adrenaline rush, I have *not* observed adrenaline infusions that were *not* marked by moments of clarity and retention.

Our time at Danny's memorial was an intense emotional experience for David. Perhaps the simultaneous and prolonged adrenaline infusion that accompanied the experience allowed him to think clearly while we were at the monument. The adrenaline may also have been a sufficient chemical marker to imprint his brain with memories of our experience for two days following the actual event.

Playing devil's advocate, my friend Michael asked me, "So what? Do you propose scaring people into moments of clarity? What's the value of your observation?"

For me, the value is in broadening my understanding of David's experience, because my compassion for him always expands in proportion to my understanding of his reality.

Meeting Terry at the Airport

Five days have passed. Terry is returning from Chicago, and we're on our way to meet her at the airport. Since David awoke eight hours ago, we have been talking about Terry's return. For these eight hours he has been asking me the same half-dozen questions without seeming to hear my answers.

"Where are we going?" David asks.

"We're going to meet Terry at the airport."

"Who is Terry?"

"Terry is your wife."

"I'm married?"

"Yes, you are."

(Looks like we're into another round of "Who's on First?")

"Does this Terry know we're married?" he laughs.

"She certainly does. You've been married to her for sixty-two years."

"No kidding … sixty-two years? You must think I'm crazy! Where is Terry now? Why did she leave me?"

"She didn't leave you. She went to Chicago for five days on an architectural tour."

"She should have taken me with her."

"That would have been wonderful, David, but you no longer travel. Your doctor and longtime friend, Abe Kauvar, has advised against your traveling, so you stayed home here in Denver while Terry went on this short trip."

"Well, okay … but where does Terry live?"

"The two of you live together, here in Denver, at 18 Windsong Lane."

"This is crazy! God, I hope I recognize her. Gee, we've been driving a hell of a long time! Where are you taking me?"

"We're going to meet Terry at the airport."

"Who is Terry?"

"Terry is your wife."

"My wife? You're crazy! I'm not married ... am I?"

"You *are* married, David. You and Terry recently celebrated your sixty-second wedding anniversary."

David turns and looks out the car window. We drive in silence. Several minutes pass before he says, "I'm not worth a damn. They must have a place for people like me—a place where I'll have what I need but won't be a problem for myself and everyone else."

"There are places where retired people can live and receive wonderful care, David, but you're not ready for that sort of arrangement. Oh, David, look at the magnificent sunset!"

"Wow! Spectacular! By the way, Dear, where are we going?"

WHEN TERRY LEAVES for several days, David is initially angry, then anxious, confused, and eventually accepting. This sequence usually plays out over a twelve-hour period. I have learned that David copes more successfully during the first twelve hours of Terry's absence if we stay home, don't have visitors, and amuse ourselves in simple ways.

During this transition time I make all of the decisions. When I give David options, he demonstrates his frustration by responding negatively. For twelve hours I eliminate opportunities for him to use me as a target for his resentment.

If I suggest, "David would you like to look at this book with me?" his answer will be "No!"

Instead I say, "For months, I've been wanting to look at this book on South American folk art. I'm going to take a few minutes right now to do it. I'd love to have your company, David, if you have the time."

I begin looking at the book alone, commenting on what I see. Usually David joins me. If he prefers to sit in the sunshine and doze, that's fine too. My only goal is to facilitate a placid, first twelve hours.

When Terry is away, another thing I notice—whether she is on an extended trip or out for an evening—David consistently punishes her when she calls or returns. He tells her he hasn't done anything fun, the food is mediocre. We could have been out hang gliding or dining with the queen. David would try to convince Terry that life during her absence was not just uneventful, but bleak.

This behavior is especially easy to detect in the context of a phone call. From our end of the line I hear, "Oh, not much. No, nothing really. Only so-so. I guess so. Probably not. I doubt that I'll feel like it."

He hangs up and says, "Now, what are we going to do? Do we need to make a dinner reservation? Should we plan on a movie after we eat? My God, it looks like a gorgeous day out there!"

Terry is in a hard spot. Though she cherishes David, her survival depends on having time away from him. She faithfully calls David, because she doesn't want him to feel abandoned. But talking with him daily and patiently giving the lengthy explanations that he requires definitely detract from her vacation.

By chance, one time when Terry is away, I discover a solution that is good for both Terry and David: voice mail. We are out when she calls. She leaves a cheerful, detailed message for David. When we return, David listens to the message and is thrilled. I offer to play it for him again. For ten minutes I replay the message. David hangs up feeling loved and satisfied. I save the message.

Next morning, David complains that he hasn't heard from Terry. I say, "Oh yes, David, she left a message for you!" Again for ten minutes I replay the message with the same positive result as the previous night.

This one message sustains David throughout Terry's entire absence. An added benefit: Terry's voice is available to David whenever he needs to hear it, not just when Terry's schedule permits a phone call.

4

Hitting Our Stride

Christmas at the Botanic Gardens

It's Christmastime. David and Terry have agreed to go with me one evening to see the holiday lights at the Denver Botanic Gardens. I know they will enjoy this exceptional display of artistry, which is not the standard seasonal cliché but a shimmering unity of color and meticulous design. We are bundled against crackling cold. David is expansively chipper, contemplating nighttime adventure.

When we arrive at the gardens, I excuse myself and return with the wheelchair I have reserved. David is insulted and protests loudly that he "won't be pushed around in a damned wheelchair by women!" Matter-of-factly, I tell him he has no choice and is making a spectacle of himself. I guide him firmly into the chair. Away we roll. The wheelchair is never mentioned again.

For the next hour David is mesmerized by the dazzling splendor. We pass through sparkling canyons created by towering, light-blanketed specimens of horticulture. In contrast there are broad, distant vistas that create the illusion of fireworks frozen against the inky winter sky. There is something ethereal and pleasantly disorienting about our experience. The darkness of night is a three-dimensional, floating canvas without perimeters. Neither we nor the lights seem anchored.

Enveloped by the warmth inside our coats, yet stung by the biting, crystalline-cold air around us, we glide on. David is awed, and his dear face glows blissfully in the reflected holiday light. A constant appreciative murmur hums from the other guests who mill along the garden walkways. This hushed buzz is punctuated by

David's enthusiastic exclamations of "The most …" "The best …" "Fan*tastic*!" "Spectacular!" "What a knockout!"

Back in the car, David announces that he isn't ready to go home, so we drive downtown to see the light display at the Civic Center. Abundant, well-placed lights artfully enhance the classic architectural detail of the massive City and County Building. Enormous columns and arches have been transformed into vibrant, gossamer transparencies of color.

One moment David effuses over this stunning display. The next moment he looks away from the splendor of the lights and sees the chaotic, plastic hodgepodge that clutters the imposing entry to this grand structure. Yellowing snowmen serve as tired sentinels near Santa's shanty of a workshop. Elves decked in fading Christmas red vie for attention with the humble, the royal, and the wise who pay homage at the nearby manger. Reindeer and angels jockey on high for airspace. David withdraws his earlier unequivocal endorsement and pronounces the jumble "an embarrassment."

We continue on to lower downtown and Union Station, then back up Seventeenth Street to Broadway. Energized by the holiday shine and bustle, David craves more adventure.

I know of a street in a nearby residential neighborhood where every house on the block is festooned with lights. As we turn onto this street David cheers, "Wow! Wow! Wow! This is the most spectacular, fantastic thing I have ever seen in my entire life!" Typically, David expresses his enthusiasm in superlatives.

When he suggests that we stop somewhere for refreshments, Terry says, "Enough!" and we turn toward home. David's bliss has been worth every bit of effort invested in this night ramble.

Paulino Gardens

Visiting Paulino Gardens is a springtime ritual for David and me. Paulino's is an enormous greenhouse and nursery that offers an opulence of botanical exotica. In May the vast and colorful array of bedding plants looks kaleidoscopic. The moisture in the air is light and cool. The fragrance of damp earth and flowers is aromatherapy par excellence. Just walking through the door of Paulino's invigorates us.

David pushes our shopping cart as we move along broad pathways, reveling in the sensory extravaganza. Simultaneously, we spy a vivid, magenta bougainvillea, striking with its rich profusion of blossoms against unusually dark green foliage. We eye each other knowingly. This fine specimen won't spend another night in a greenhouse!

The bougainvillea is a frill. Our main mission at Paulino's is to purchase bedding plants for my garden and flowers and herbs for all my summer pots. Having huddled head-to-head over our many choices, we finish our shopping and move into the checkout line. Grandiosely, David announces that he will be paying for everything—a sizable tab.

"How generous of you, David, but I need to pay for all of this myself. These plants are for my garden," I explain.

Agitated, he answers, "Well, Goddamn it, something's wrong if I can't buy you a nice present once in a while!"

"David! How about a birthday present when the time comes?" I suggest.

Now David is shouting, "I may not live that long! This is *my* money, and *you* can't tell me how to spend it. Get the hell out of my way and let me pay."

Stepping close to him, I speak softly into his ear. "Thank you, David. I accept your beautiful gift. You are thoughtful and generous."

"Okay," he responds in a calm, flat voice. "Glad you see it my way," he mumbles through the beginning flicker of a grin.

On our way home, I stop at an ATM for cash. At the first discreet opportunity, I slip the money to Terry with the brief explanation, "David needed the satisfaction of paying for my bedding plants, so I agreed. This covers it."

I've just perpetuated a public lie.

Movies

David, a longtime movie enthusiast, still sees himself as someone who enjoys all of the latest cinematic attractions. Frequently he suggests that we see a movie together. The reality is that David's condition now prevents his following even the simplest story line. Often a movie's language and aggressive action initially upset him. "This is terrible! Can you believe what they're saying? I think we should leave, don't you?" But, unable to understand what he is seeing, and lulled by the theater's darkness, David soon falls asleep. When occasionally he rouses, he is always confused and agitated, disoriented by the darkness, unfamiliar sounds, and strange surroundings. In no way does going to a movie contribute to his well-being.

I never take him to a movie so I can have a break. When I'm with David, I'm with David. I see movies on my own time. If I need a break, I tell him I need a break. I set him up in his favorite chair, preferably in the sunshine. He is content to look at a magazine or newspaper. Now I am free for a time to read, write a letter, or make a phone call. Usually David falls asleep, but when he awakens he is serene—free from anxiety. In familiar surroundings there is no need for several hours of reorientation.

One exception to my movie policy: I rent videos of old musicals. The first time we rent a musical, David falls asleep. I think: *Well, this is a bomb.* But continuing to sit next to him, I realize that he is 100 percent content. Something clicks for me: *The only reason I'm here is to facilitate David's contentment.*

Not particularly interested in the movie, I pick up a magazine. When the next musical number begins, I decide to nudge David to see if he is interested. He is very interested. Accompanied by the actors on the screen, we sing like veteran karaoke crooners. Song complete, David is pleased with himself, but within five minutes he is again confused by the movie and falls asleep. I sit close to him, reading my book, giving him the comfort of human warmth and presence until it's time for the next song.

So David doesn't actually watch movies, he participates in "sing 'n' doze" sessions. The only criterion by which I measure an activity's success is the level of David's contentment as he participates in his own way.

She's Our Enemy

Terry and David have a new dog, Buddy. Terry has hired a dour, middle-aged woman named Loraine to walk him every night. Loraine and Buddy are out on their walk when I arrive to stay with David. Terry will be attending a play.

Terry leaves. David is angry, confused, and sad that he has been excluded from her plans.

For a few minutes David vents his frustration on me. I invite him to join me in the kitchen while I cook our dinner. He declines, choosing instead to sit morosely in the living room, staring blankly into space.

Loraine returns with Buddy, and, as is her nightly habit, she mixes a martini for herself and settles in to watch *Jeopardy!*

From the living room David shouts, "Turn that off! It's bothering me." Typically genial and easygoing, David is not given to petulant outbursts. I see his behavior as an indicator of how deeply troubled he is over his exclusion from Terry's social plans.

With an edge to her voice Loraine calls back, "*No*, I'm watching it!"

I am stunned by Loraine's response, but I have no authority over her. I ask Loraine to at least turn down the volume. She complies. Moments later David yells again, "I said turn it off!"

Loraine ignores him. He goes upstairs to his room.

When dinner is ready I look for David and find him sitting in his dark bedroom. Only my best finessing persuades him to join me for dinner downstairs. But he sees Loraine from the top of the stairs. Pointing at her, he shrieks, "There she is! I don't like that girl! Get her out of here! She's our enemy!" He won't go down a single step.

Loraine is unresponsive, seemingly unconcerned by David's agitation and anxiety. But soon *Jeopardy!* ends. She finishes the last of her martini and leaves.

Even after Loraine's departure, David refuses to come down for dinner. He puts on his nightshirt and goes to bed. I eat alone and clean up the kitchen.

Around 8:45 P.M., David appears, fully dressed. "What are the chances a guy could get some breakfast around here?" he asks pleasantly.

I reheat his dinner. He eats it with gusto.

Protocol, Savvy, and Intelligence

David has a sense of propriety uncommon in this day of casual dress, casual talk, and liberated women. Just as he worries about my spending the night at his house when Terry is away, he feels like a failure if he is unable to open a door for a woman. He is most comfortable if he has the opportunity to change into a sport coat for dinner, and somewhat annoyed by "men who dine in shirtsleeves."

Proper introductions are also important to David. In a grocery checkout line, I call our clerk by name—having just read her name tag. She and I visit superficially as she rings up our purchases. Leaving, I say, "Thank you, Rose. Be good to yourself."

David is indignant with me. "Why didn't you introduce me to your friend? The two of you were so glad to see each other you just forgot about me!"

I AM TAKING David to his weekly lunch with a group of his friends who call themselves the ROMEOs (Retired Old Men Eating Out). En route to the restaurant, David quizzes me repeatedly about how the introductions will go. Many times during our few minutes of travel, he is mortified that he doesn't remember my name, and fearful that he will be unable to gracefully introduce me. I know all of the ROMEOs. There will be no need for introductions. My telling

David this does not pacify him. He is consumed by anxiety—afraid of being inadequate. To calm his frenzy I pull over, write my name on a slip of paper, and put it into his shirt pocket. We drive on and every time David mentions introductions, I remind him of the paper with my name on it. He retrieves the paper, reads my name, and his fear dissolves.

If introductions were actually required, David would not remember to look for my name in his pocket. No matter. He will breeze through our arrival at the restaurant, my name tucked into his pocket like the feather in Baby Dumbo's trunk.

DAVID CLINGS TO THE old protocols that have served him well, though he often lacks the savvy to integrate them appropriately. Yet he perceives other nuances—a tone of voice, a glance, a facial expression, and sometimes even body language—with disarming insight. There is no predicting what David will understand, or when his brilliant flashes of recognition will occur. I value this element of uncertainty. It spices our relationship, keeps me alert, and prevents me from sliding into a dismissive attitude toward him. My mission is to be observant, to notice David's moments of brilliance, and to affirm these for him.

From the moment my two children were born, I assumed they were both geniuses—trapped in bodies that didn't fully support their intelligence. I view David similarly. I have no way of knowing the breadth and depth of his intelligence. I know it is broader and deeper than many might guess. I prefer to err on the side of believing David understands more rather than less. If I am wrong, what's the harm?

There are times when David has difficulty completing a coherent sentence. Developing original ideas or abstract concepts is usually challenging for him. His language skills are most likely to deteriorate when he ventures into areas of creative thinking. But given the opportunity to react spontaneously to the moment, David shines. He may comment articulately on the gathering storm clouds that suddenly obscure the sun. But he will likely have difficulty expressing the more abstract concept that, as we approach winter, darkness comes earlier in the day.

Once recognized for his exceptional mind, David is sadly aware of his intellectual losses. We talk about it daily. I feed him the hackneyed "Yesterday is gone, tomorrow is not yet here, today is all we have." He's not buying it, and good for him. David still has spunk enough to resist what he perceives as a gloss-over.

Breakfast in Italy

One morning when I arrive, Terry has already left to do errands. David is sitting on the living room sofa, asleep. I sit down next to him and nudge him toward consciousness. Groggily he tries to focus.

"Oh hello, Dear," he mumbles, squinting out of his fog. "I don't understand why I'm so tired this morning. I can't stay awake. Of course, I ate breakfast in Italy, and the trip home was pretty long. I'm not sure that would explain my drowsiness, though."

"David, maybe you were *dreaming* of Italy just now. Could that be?" I ask.

"Well, no. I think I *was* in Italy."

"As far as I know, you've been here in Denver the whole time, David. Decades ago you traveled to Italy, but you haven't left Denver, Colorado, in years. But here's something to think about. Many people believe in something called astral projection, or time travel. I've read a book that says as people age, they are more likely to have time-travel experiences."

"What exactly would that mean, Dear?" he asks before I can explain.

"My understanding of the subject is limited, David, but basically I think it means that your body stays in Denver, while your mind, or maybe your spirit, travels freely—say, to Italy."

"No kidding! That's fascinating. And Italy! Funny you should mention Italy—I had breakfast in Italy just this morning!"

Terry Attends a Funeral

On short notice Terry calls to say she will be attending a funeral. She asks if I can check in with David while she is gone. She plans to leave at 2:00. I arrive at 1:55 and find that she has left early. The front door is standing open. David is crumpled on the floor of the entry hall, tangled in a mass of thick winter coats and scarves. The coat closet is empty, its entire contents having recently cushioned his fall.

David is crying. "Oh my God, Darling!" he sobs. "Thank God you're here! I can't get up, and I have to meet Terry at a funeral. I was trying to decide which coat to wear. I lost my balance and fell. I've been here like this for hours."

Within five minutes the scene is restored to normal; David is on his feet, unscathed; the incident is forgotten. I feel certain that, had he not fallen, he would have soon chosen a coat and set out through the open front door "for the funeral."

I am more determined than ever that David must not be left alone.

YEARS LATER, Terry reflects on this episode and tells me, "It was hard for me to admit that David had reached the point when he couldn't be left alone. It hurt me for him. Somehow I felt I was betraying David—letting him down—if I admitted that he couldn't be alone in his own home."

Sick Dog

Terry is out. David is pacing. I am preparing lunch. From the dining room comes an alarmed "Hey! What's this?"

I find David standing in excrement and vomit on an Oriental rug! Buddy, the dog, has been sick. The soles of David's shoes are covered with the dreck, but worse, he has accomplished many tracking revolutions around the dining room table.

Buddy has left *his* sorry footprints across the dining room rug, the hardwood floor, and another Oriental carpet in the living room where he is still retching.

I help David out of his shoes and serve him his lunch at the breakfast table, around the corner from crisis central.

The cleanup is slow going. As I work I realize that the entire mess is laden with peanuts. Despite frequent instruction to the contrary, David has generously shared his snacks with Buddy.

What About Me?

Mostly David views me as his ally, but there are times when he is overwhelmed by the frustrations of his situation, and he lashes out at me.

Angry that Terry is out for the morning, David turns on me. "You are always butting in around here. If it weren't for you, Terry would spend more time with me. She'd be here right now!"

"You're right, David—perceptive as usual. Terry *would* spend more time with you if I weren't here. But Terry is eighty-four and you're ninety-one. Terry realizes that she needs help managing things around here so the two of you can continue living comfortably. I'm here to help."

David glimpses only a thin slice of reality, lacking full understanding of his limitations and how these limitations define the big picture of our three, interwoven lives.

When Terry is home, David notices that she is eager to engage with me—Terry needs support too. Regularly, David insinuates himself into our conversations with "Hey! What about *me*? Why isn't anyone paying attention to *me*?"

Terry and I don't intentionally exclude David, but our interactions quickly and naturally evolve beyond his comprehension and ability to keep pace with us. Terry and I might as well be speaking in code. David is effectively excluded.

5

Some Days Are
Better Than Others

Two Cathedrals and a Rotunda

David is in a state of rare and sustained lucidity. We are on our way to lunch at the Denver Art Museum when David points to St. John's Cathedral, commenting, "I've always wanted to see inside that place." St. John's occupies an entire city block near downtown Denver. With just enough advance notice to accomplish a detour, I careen into the cathedral parking lot.

The month is January. Workers are dismantling Christmas decorations: lights, wreaths, garland swags, and a towering blue spruce tree. Unnoticed, we enter the sanctuary.

David, observant as always, is awestruck by the cathedral's majestic immensity; the brilliance, abundance, and intricacy of its stained glass; and the Old World richness of its dark, patinaed wood. The stained glass of St. John's, designed by some of the world's most accomplished craftsmen, is exceptional and widely revered. One window, designed by Tiffany of New York, dates back to 1890. We walk the long side aisles of the nave, craning our necks painfully, trying to read the words of memoriam beneath each massive window.

After fifteen minutes of window-gazing, I sense that David's interest is flagging. I am a breath away from suggesting we go to lunch when we find a window dedicated to Edwin George Arkins, who died at age thirty-five, on August 4, 1905, the day after David was born. David is suddenly electrified, driven. This experience has become personal. Accompanied by the tune of our growling stomachs, we pay homage at every remaining stained-glass window in the cathedral.

David leaves St. John's with a deep sense of accomplishment. He has completed something important.

Walking back to the car, David stops the first person we see in the parking lot. He tells the unsuspecting stranger about a young man who "died on August 4, 1905, the day after *my own birthday!*" With conviction he adds, "Do yourself a favor. Take a few minutes to look at those windows and read those inscriptions."

As David chatters enthusiastically at my elbow, I wonder about the transient nature of our existence. An old man has just paid tribute, out of sincere respect, certainly, but perhaps with a fleeting thought to his own future—a future when another old man, maybe not yet born, may linger to read an inscription honoring a remarkable man, David Saul Touff, born August 3, 1905, in Freeland, Michigan. I am convinced that on some level, David feels he has picked up a thread of life and woven it into the continuum.

After lunch, David is eager to see another cathedral. Scrapping our plans to stroll around the art museum, we decide to visit the Cathedral of the Immaculate Conception, host cathedral to Pope John Paul when he visited Denver in 1993. This Gothic Revival structure, completed in 1912, is noted for its 210-foot, twin bell spires, a city landmark. Inside we find altars of Italian marble and hand-carved pews of golden oak. A sixty-eight-foot-high vaulted ceiling canopies a sanctuary that seats 1,500 people. Bas-relief sculptures depicting the Stations of the Cross adorn the walls.

David is intrigued by these sculptures, and I am intrigued by David—this frail yet dignified Jewish man beside me, open-minded and life-embracing enough at age ninety-two to reverently enter a Catholic church with appreciation for a belief system foreign to his own. He suggests that we each light a candle and pause for a moment of contemplation before we leave. Momentarily I tense at the thought of a delay; I'm ready to move on. Then I catch myself: *Why am I in such a hurry? Habit I guess. I am only here to support David, and we have all afternoon.*

We light our candles and observe separate, silent moments. I spend *my* moment being thankful for David and for the opportunity I've been given to learn from him.

AT THE OUTSET of our relationship, David's slow crawl was a challenge for me. It's likely that back in the early days of knowing him I would have said, "David, let's not take time to light candles." But gradually, I am adjusting my pace to match his.

Perhaps David's natural inclination has always been to appreciate his surroundings and the present moment, but age and dementia have slowed his pace and allow him to be even more alert to the details of his environment. David, the "Be Here Now" poster boy! By example, he consistently reminds me to be receptive to life outside of my scheduled focus. And traveling slowly, I have the time to notice what David needs most: a loving, attentive, human presence—a person who will come to him with acceptance and participate with him just as he is at any given moment. Although I understand that the present is our only arena for experience (the past and future being abstractions), I have also begun to suspect that pop psychology has overglorified and oversimplified the value of the "precious present."

Being locked exclusively in the present, denied full access to the learning and fulfillment of his past, unable to create aspirations for his future, David has been robbed of his wholeness and the fullness of his life. Surely, the ideal must be to find a balance—to acknowledge that our past and our future enable us to maximize our present.

OUT IN THE SUNSHINE AGAIN, we see the state capitol building in the near distance. David is excited by the lure of the gleaming gold dome. We nourish the parking meter and walk the intervening blocks to our next adventure. David has been inside the capitol on many occasions, but one of the gifts of dementia is that all things become new.

Squinting at the dome, David exclaims, "My God, it looks like real gold! How do they keep it so shiny?"

"It *is* real gold, David," I tell him.

"You've got to be wrong about that."

"No, seriously, David, in the early 1900s the dome was plated with 24-karat gold to commemorate the discovery of gold by the early Colorado pioneers."

"Well, that doesn't sound right. It would take a hell of a lot of gold to do that job. But I'm not going to argue with you."

"David, I'll tell you a supposedly true story about the dome. Years ago, some enterprising fellow came up with a scheme for stealing the gold off the dome. After he was caught, the powers that be decided the dome should be painted to thwart further attempts to steal the gold. Years passed while the gold lay unappreciated under layers of paint. In time, it was decided the gold dome is part of Colorado's unique heritage, and the paint was removed."

"All right, enough gold talk. You seem to believe it's gold, so I'll go along with it. Let's go."

The afternoon is bright, brittle-cold, Colorado-in-January. At the base of the steep marble stairs leading to the north entrance of the capitol, I question the wisdom of our endeavor. David will not be dissuaded. For ten minutes we teeter tentatively up the icy stairs. Usually undaunted, I am apprehensive, and even suggest that we turn back. I am thinking not only of the challenge of making it to the top, but of the later, colder, darker hazard of descent. David is committed. For him to turn back would be tantamount to giving up on Mt. Everest twenty feet from the summit. Sir Edmund Hillary would have admired David's resolve.

Once inside the capitol, an august, neoclassical structure of marble and white granite, we go first to the central rotunda. There we look straight up into the top of the dome that rises 150 feet above us. David is euphoric to the point of giddiness. Taking in the enormous, gilded grandeur, he insists on seeing every area open to the public.

Eventually we stand under the west portico, protected from the cold, warming in the afternoon sun as we survey the panorama of Civic Center Park far below. In the forest of winter-barren trees lie large plazas, two amphitheaters, and a mosaic of dormant gardens, all connected by a labyrinth of broad walkways alive with people who, from our lofty perspective, are Lilliputian. Four blocks away, the arcing City and County Building defines the park's western perimeter. Fringing our view is the contemporary geometry of skyscrapers.

"Where are we, Dear?" David asks.

"We're in Denver, David."

"No, kidding! Denver? My God, I had no idea! Denver is bigger than New York!"

"Well, as impressive as it is from this spot, David, Denver is still a relatively small city. It's home to us, though, and large or small, we like it here."

"You're damn right about that! Just look at that view!" he says with a sweep of his arm. "Spectacular! A real knockout! Where did you say we are, Dear?"

"We're in Denver, David. Look to your left, over there on the other side of the park, you can see the Denver Art Museum. You and Terry served on the museum's board of directors."

"Wow! We did that?" David asks, delighted.

"That and a lot more, David. This is your city. You've left your mark here. Just beyond those skyscrapers over there is where May D&F, under your presidential leadership, built the store designed by the world-renowned architect I. M. Pei. Pei is the same architect who designed the glass pyramid at the entrance of the Louvre in Paris. Your building had an amazing parabola roof and for years was a landmark in Denver."

"Keep talking, Dear, this is tremendously exciting!"

Descending from where we stand is another long, formidable flight of stairs. At the base of these stairs is a monument. David believes the monument commemorates the Civil War, but he wants to know why there is a Civil War monument in Colorado. He insists that we investigate.

Venturing down the stairs with David is not an option, and emphatically I say so. He looks defeated, pathetic. Without thinking,

I offer to go down alone on a reconnaissance mission. David brightens. Too late I realize that my solo excursion will leave him unsteady, unreliable, and precariously perched—alone at the top of the stairs. To turn away now will be anticlimactic; to forge ahead may bring disaster. For a more prudent woman, the choice would be clear. I go down to investigate.

David was right. The statue is of a Civil War cavalryman. The monument, unveiled on July 24, 1909, honors the Colorado (then Jefferson Territory) soldiers and unknown men who fought and died in the Civil War.

I wonder: *How does David know the statue is a Civil War monument? Is he remembering it from a previous visit? Can he actually identify the soldier's uniform?* If I ask him right now what he ate for lunch, he will ask me if he has *eaten* lunch. Turning to look up at him, small and fragile at the top of the stairs, I doubt that David even has a geographic context for this moment in time.

Hurrying, I climb back to David. He waits, statuelike himself, having taken seriously my admonition, "While I'm down there, don't breathe, don't wiggle!"

"David, you were right!" I breathlessly congratulate him, then describe the details of the monument. As I talk, I notice that David is standing in front of a bronze plaque inscribed with the full text of the Gettysburg Address. I begin reading: "'Four score and seven years ago, our fathers brought forth on this continent a new nation, conceived in liberty …'"

Without hesitation, in the booming voice of an orator, David picks up in midsentence, "'and dedicated to the proposition that all men are created equal. Now we are engaged in a great civil war …'"

We speak in unison: David reciting from memory, I, reading as best I can, my eyes blurred with tears, voice choked with emotion. David continues, strong to the end: "'… that government of the people, by the people, for the people shall not perish from the earth.'" Passersby look our way and surely wonder. I am learning another valuable lesson in releasing my inhibitions.

Back inside we pause to look at the Boettcher Water Murals on the walls of the circular room that surrounds the capitol's grand staircase. Dedicated to Colorado philanthropist Charles Boettcher, these eight striking murals depict western, water-related scenes from ancient to contemporary times. Denver artist Allen Tupper True, an elected fellow to Britain's Royal Society of Artists, painted them in 1940. The murals are immeasurably enhanced by the accompanying poetry of Thomas Hornsby Ferril, Colorado's premier poet laureate, whom Carl Sandburg called "the great poet of the West." This sample of Ferril's poetry focuses on the role of water in the development of the West. I read aloud his introductory verses:

> *Here is a land where life is written in water,*
> *The West is where the water was and is,*
> *Father and son of old, mother and daughter,*
> *Following Rivers up immensities*
> *Of range and desert, thirsting the sundown ever,*
> *Crossing a hill to climb a hill still drier,*
> *Naming tonight a City by some River*
> *A different name from last night's camping fire.*
>
> *Look to the green within the mountain cup,*
> *Look to the prairie parched for water lack,*
> *Look to the sun that pulls the oceans up,*
> *Look to the cloud that gives the oceans back,*
> *Look to your heart and may your wisdom grow*
> *To power of lightning and to peace of snow.**

"Wow! I like that last part. Read it again," David urges, and I repeat the last stanza.

Beneath the murals is inscribed more of Ferril's poetry. I read aloud:

---

*"Trial by Time," copyright © 1971 by Thomas Hornsby Ferril. Reprinted by permission of HarperCollins Publishers Inc.

Men shall behold the water in the sky
And count the seasons by the living grasses.

Then shall the river namers track the sunset,
Singing the long song to the Shining Mountains.

Here shall the melting snows renew the oxen,
Here firewood is and here shall men build cities.

Water shall sluice the gold yellow as leaves
That fall from silver trees on silent hills.

And men shall fashion glaciers into greenness
And harvest April rivers in the autumn.

Deep in the earth where roots of willows drank
Shall aqueducts be laid to nourish cities.

Water the lightning gave shall give back lightning
And men shall store the lightning for their use.

Beyond the sundown is tomorrow's wisdom,
Today is going to be long long ago.*

Without a pause, David turns to me and says:

"And I have left so very few tomorrows
That will become my own long long ago."

David has just added his own original couplet that perfectly matches
Ferril's tone and cadence. Speechless, tears brimming again, I turn to
David. He takes my hand and says, "My God, who else in the world
would bring me here to this marvelous place, read these things to me,
and stand here crying for me? You're terrific, Darling! Let's get out of
here and go home."

---

*"Trial by Time," copyright © 1971 by Thomas Hornsby Ferril. Reprinted by permission of
HarperCollins Publishers Inc.

The day has been idyllic. We emerge from the mammoth cocoon of the capitol, and I return to real time, realizing that we must hurry to avoid a parking ticket.

As he often does when my energy surges, David stops, rooted to the spot. "Wait a minute," he commands, gripping my arm and gesturing broadly. "Just look at that spectacular sunset! Look at the lines of the tree branches silhouetted against the blazing sky."

"David, you are remarkable to notice these things and so poetic in your expression!" I exclaim.

Like a kid caught trying to act mature beyond his years, David grins timidly. "It's not really me," he says. "Terry has taught me everything I know about beauty."

We stand shivering together, watching the paling sunset. Our meter has expired, but it is not our day for a ticket.

FIFTEEN MINUTES LATER WE return to David's house and are welcomed by Terry. Eager to share with her the details of our incredible day, I prompt, "David, tell Terry what we found in St. John's Cathedral."

Looking blank, he shakes his head.

"Well, let's tell her about our visit to the capitol," I encourage.

Confused and anxious, David mumbles, "I'm sorry, Dear, but I don't know what you're talking about."

The day has been a mirage. Or has it? Must something be remembered for it to be significant, meaningful, real? The day was *vividly* real as we experienced it together. As I recall it now, it is real again. But if I too forget our day together, the time we shared will never be diminished.

Our day of cathedral hopping and capitol touring leaves an indelible impression on me. I think of that day often and sense that in some essential way it has left me changed.

THE CRACKLE OF JANUARY ICE IS eventually replaced by warm spring rain. One late afternoon in May as I sort through my mail I become vaguely aware that the light outside is odd—eerie, surreal. I look out the window to see that the world is enveloped in an ethereal, golden glow. Stepping outside, I feel I have been transported to another realm. Everything around me seems altered by this exquisite, velvet, butter-light. The atmosphere is heavy with moisture. The air blankets my skin. I feel expansive, lighter, momentarily transformed. I stand, breathing deeply as the magical light washes over me.

The sun falls lower in the sky, the light shifts, the moment passes. I step back inside. I feel transformed, and this feeling stays with me long into the evening.

This one experience probably won't alter my life. But I have discovered that welcoming the opportunity of the moment enhances the quality of my days and, I believe, ultimately the quality of my life.

I recall my January day with David and begin to understand what had seemed mysterious to me before. I am beginning to open to the same willingness to experience life around me that I have been observing in David. In the process of supporting him, not only have I become more attentive and receptive to the full spectrum of his human experience—his enthusiasm as well as his despair, his perceptiveness as well as his rage and terror—I am becoming more immersed in my own humanity.

Being an observant person by nature, I likely would have noticed the golden light as I looked through my mail, but without David's influence, I probably would not have paused for five minutes to step outside into a breathtaking world.

Riding the Light Rail

Adventures with David are becoming more challenging. He now requires much more physical support from me. Even though he uses his cane, he leans heavily on me when we walk. This new demand exhausts me, but without my support David trips and staggers. Recently he has fallen several times.

Further, David's spatial and social awarenesses seem dramatically diminished. Routinely, he stumbles into other pedestrians with no apparent sense that he may have offended. Too often his comments in public lack a forgivable, childlike charm.

So it is with some apprehension that I set out with David, one blue-sky morning in summer, to ride the light rail, a recent state-of-the-art addition to Denver. We'll ride the train to the end of the line, return to town via the same train, eat lunch, and late in the afternoon take the train back to our starting point. David is high-spirited, confident, happy to be on the road again, and clueless about our agenda, though we have discussed it unceasingly since I picked him up at his house.

David is exhilarated by the smooth and quiet train ride, our fellow passengers, and the opportunity to see Denver, his home for sixty-one years, from a new perspective. We cruise through downtown and move along toward Five Points, a predominantly black area of the inner city. The farther from downtown and the closer to Five Points we travel, the fewer white faces we see around us and the less affluent is our view from the train window.

Ever the commentator, David remarks to everyone and no one, "What I can't understand is why the city has spent millions of tax-payer dollars extending the route for this beautiful, modern train into this run-down neighborhood." I am dumbstruck. There is nothing to say. I look away from David, mortified.

The train stops. People exit. We are a minority of two.

At the next stop a white woman, a black man, and a child board the train together. David points at them. Again in a voice loud enough for too many to hear, he offers, "That's another thing I can't understand, why any white woman would ever take up with a colored man, especially one who looks like he does."

Now I am nauseated. I turn my back to David. My rage and mortification are mingled with apprehension. I sit stone-faced, mute, dreading to meet the eyes of the other passengers. We ride along in a charged silence. Reaching the end of the line, the train pauses for several minutes, then moves back toward downtown.

David leans in my direction and whispers to my back, "Are you upset with me?"

"Yes," I hiss over my shoulder. His hurt and confused expression is pitiful.

"Why?" he asks, contrite, uncomprehending.

Softening, I say, "This is not the place to discuss it, David, but everything will be okay."

By the time we reach "the place to discuss it," the moment has long passed. David has forgotten my anger. Reconstructing the episode for him would be impossible and pointless. He wouldn't understand the complexity of the story, nor would he retain anything to apply to a similar, future circumstance.

DOWNTOWN, DAVID AND I hike the Sixteenth Street Mall to LoDo. We're on our way to the Oxford Hotel for lunch. I can see that he is wilting in the high-noon sun, and I suggest that we hop the shuttle to lower downtown. David is indignant. I am a heretic. We plod on.

Having crossed the Sahara, we arrive, parched, at the Oxford Hotel. I take a quick step ahead of David to open the door for him.

"Don't open that door for me—you make me feel like an old man! No, you make me feel like no man at all. I should open the door for *you.*"

David's wanting to retain his image of himself as a chivalrous man presents me with a difficult dilemma: How to preserve his self-esteem, protect him from the embarrassment of not being able to open a too-heavy door, and pay him the respect he is due.

"Sorry, David," I offer. "Not trying to make you feel like an old man, but you *are* a few years older than I am, so when I *don't* open the door for you, I feel disrespectful."

"Well, I see what you mean, just don't make a *habit* of opening doors for me," he grins.

Years ago, David would meet friends at the Oxford for lunch. Now he asks the waitress, "Have any of the fellas been in?" These are "fellas" who retired and left downtown Denver years before our waitress was born. But David seems confident that if he persists with

names and associations, the lights will come on for our eighteen-
year-old friend, and they will discover acres of common ground.
Though young, our waitress is savvy enough to remain securely
behind the mask of her waitress character, beguiling David with
smiles and keeping the dialogue simple. Her repertoire of "Yes sir,"
"No sir," "I don't know sir" sees her through.

Ten men are seated at a nearby table. We can hear their congenial,
easy-flowing repartee. David watches intently, wistfully. He thinks
he recognizes several of the men, then decides he doesn't. Still he puzzles, "I don't understand why they don't invite me to join them."

Thoroughly engrossed with the familiar environment and his
reminiscing, David hardly notices that he is eating lunch.

On the street again, the sun is searing. I strongly urge that we
ride the shuttle back to the train. David's answer: a simple, determined, "No!"

I figure: *if he dies now, at least he'll die happy. I just hope I don't pre-
decease him.*

Reaching the train platform, I feel like I've carried David piggy-
back all the way. My head is pounding; I'm feeling resentful—questioning whether I can continue these adventures.

Triumphantly David announces, "It nearly killed me, but I
wouldn't have missed a moment of it!"

I am jolted. This simple statement from David triggers a revelation for me. It has taken me years to see the truth that has been evident from the beginning: after a lifetime of being vital and dynamic,
there are so few opportunities remaining for David to validate himself. No wonder he now feels the need to master what challenges he
has. So, he trudges up a long street in the punishing, noonday sun or
doggedly insists on paying for his friend's bedding plants.

While I'm contemplating my newfound awareness of David's
plight, he is schmoozing with a group of tourists as we all wait for the
train. He revels in the attention from this entourage.

The train arrives. One of the tourists, a tightly coifed, lavender-
haired little lady in double-knit polyester and sensible shoes, is

determined to sit with David. I sit across the aisle. Someone in the group congratulates David on his good judgment in choosing an "older, more mature woman" for his seatmate. Invigorated by the attention, he banters with the best of them as we ride along.

HOME AGAIN, David is in his room resting. I discuss the Five Points incident with Terry. She is appalled and confounded.

As one of Denver's prominent business leaders in the 1940s, 1950s, and 1960s, David was in the forefront of civil rights reform. He was the first general manager of a Denver department store to promote a black person to the position of buyer and department manager. David was not following a trend; he was breaking ground. His colleagues all recommended vehemently against such radical action. He argued that color would not be a factor in his decision; the person in question was clearly the strongest candidate. He defended an unpopular principle that he believed in, and he risked his standing in the business community. Not long after taking this stand, David was the first to employ black sales clerks.

Still, I am troubled. Though sympathetic to David, my energy and resolve are ebbing.

At the end of this bizarre day, I have dinner with Kath, a friend of mine. Railing and ranting around her kitchen, I tell the story of the day's escapade with David.

"I can't do this anymore!" I moan.

"Yeah," drawls Kath. "Looks like you'll have to quit or start wearing a nurse's uniform."

Cherry Creek Arts Festival

Our last major adventure is to the Cherry Creek Arts Festival in the summer of 1998. Terry is eager to go, but it makes her sad to think of leaving David at home. The July heat at 10:30 A.M. is already suffocating. Home is where David belongs. He doesn't understand his options, nor does he care one way or the other. After much back-and-forth, the three of us set out. Our plan is to let Terry cover all the exhibits at her usual fast pace while David and I mosey. We'll rendezvous in an hour and return home together.

David is agitated from the start—frustrated and confused about how and where "we lost Terry," overwhelmed by the crush of people.

"Where the hell did all these damn people come from?" he sneers loudly as the "damn people" stare in our direction.

"I suppose some of them are tourists; others live here in Denver, David," I answer.

"You know this is not Denver, and don't try to tell me it is!" he snaps.

Trapped by the lumbering mob, David is frantic, claustrophobic, barely able to move or see. In the rare moments when we are able to see an exhibit, he is loud and scathing in his appraisals. I feel this is grossly unfair to the artists who are dealing with potential customers. I try to coax David along. He resists. "Don't think you can force me out of here just because I don't like these god-awful paintings," he barks, sensing my agenda.

The heat is starting to affect me. I assume that David, even with his hat on, is suffering much more than I. "David, we need to find some shade," I say.

David doesn't hear me. He is having a TIA, immobilized. There is nothing to do but stand where we are in the middle of the milling crowd and let time pass. Slowly David regains his equilibrium. We make our way to a partially shaded windowsill and sit.

The car is three blocks away; I dread the walk. Eventually we set out. If David was difficult and disoriented before, he is a zombie now. Two snails on hot pavement, we inch miserably back to the car. We meet Terry and return home.

I am finished! I will not facilitate another adventure of this sort. I feel angry for allowing myself to be persuaded to do something that I feared, from the outset, was ill-advised.

6

A New Phase

Changing Expectations

I continue with David, but the goals of our outings are less lofty. Often we go to a deli for takeout and eat lunch at my house. This gives David the sense that he has been somewhere and relieves me of dealing with the challenges of public interaction. Still, there are pitfalls.

One day we arrive at the deli to pick up an order I have phoned in. There are no parking spaces. We circle. A space opens up around the corner from the deli. David has been nodding off. He says he's tired and refuses to leave the car. Subdued as he is, I am certain he won't wander away. But I am worried about leaving him in the summer heat. Choosing from unacceptable options, I pull the emergency brake, leave the engine and air conditioner running, lock the car, and race to the deli. Four minutes later I am back. David is asleep. I have a parking ticket for leaving the car running "unattended"!

My devising new ways to cope with David's mounting deficits will not eliminate the stress of caring for him. The stress will only change, and there will be plenty of it.

Grocery Shopping

Although David is having difficulty walking, most days he irritably objects to using his walker. But the less he walks, the more his walking deteriorates. The challenge is finding a way for him to walk without his walker.

Grocery shopping is a great solution—mostly. Imagining grocery shopping with David, I see aisles of smooth and level terrain that will replace uneven, hazardous sidewalks. I envision the walker that will be waiting for us, disguised as a shopping cart.

Just inside the supermarket door for our first shopping endeavor, I eagerly grab the nearest cart.

"David, if you toss your cane into the basket, you can push the cart for us while we shop."

He balks, "I'm not going to use this goddamned walker in front of all these people!"

"It's not a walker, David, it's a shopping cart," I try to reason as people sidle around us at the entrance.

"I know exactly what it is! I'm not touching it!" he argues loudly.

"David, look around. Every shopper here, young or old, is using an identical cart. One of us has to push the cart so we'll have a place to put our groceries. If you're unwilling to push it, I will. I was hoping you'd help me."

David relents. He is supported and stabilized by the cart. There is a bonus I haven't foreseen: if I am walking in front, I can quicken our pace by subtly pulling the cart.

Steadily, briskly, we glide along. David enjoys maneuvering the cart and having a responsible role in something meaningful. The downside: David has his own shopping "needs."

"Hey, wait a minute! What's your hurry? Terry will want this," he insists, clanging a large aluminum roasting pan into the cart.

"David, here is Terry's shopping list. This roasting pan is not on the list. Terry has plenty of pans at home. She won't want us to buy an extra pan."

"I know Terry needs this. She just forgot to put it on the list."

"Terry doesn't even use large roasting pans anymore, David. She definitely won't need this."

"What makes you think *you* know what Terry needs and I *don't* know?"

Reasoning is not working here. I have no ready answer that will accomplish my purpose and allow David to save face. It's my turn to relent.

"Well, maybe you're right, David. After all, you live with Terry and I don't. Maybe we'd better take that pan."

We move down the aisle. Too soon I hear, "Hey, look at this! I've been looking all over for this!" I turn to see David brandishing a can of red shoe polish like a trophy. The roasting pan standoff has already taught me that David needs the satisfaction of "shopping."

I don't flinch. "Great, David! I guess it's your lucky day. We were moving pretty fast, but you were still sharp enough to spot the red shoe polish! Toss it into the cart. We need to wrap it up here and get home to Terry. It's time for lunch."

TO ACCOMMODATE DAVID'S SHOPPING, I have learned to put a hand basket into our cart. When we finish shopping, I find the longest checkout line. Gathering all the unnecessary merchandise into the hand basket I say, "David, I realize we don't need these things after all. Will you please hold our place in line while I quickly return these items to the shelves?" David has forgotten which items he chose. He is unaware that all of the things I return are his selections.

Hurriedly restocking the shelves, I employ my "mother's eye" to see that David is still in line and not ready to check out. Holding our place in line seems to give him a sense of purpose and independence.

So, David has his exercise, enjoys being a consumer, feels useful, and the marketing is accomplished in the process. But by letting David "shop" and returning his selections to the shelves, I am supporting another public lie. I reason that a confrontation in the aisle of the grocery store serves no purpose and will embarrass us both.

Cruisin' 'n' Croonin'

David has entered another challenging phase of his decline. Given the opportunity, he will sleep in a chair for most of the day. The intolerable result of his daytime vegetating is his nighttime wakefulness. Another development is his increased level of anxiety.

Often when we are out he tirelessly repeats, "Where are you taking me? You'd better take me home now. Does Terry know we're together?"

It is a temptation to let David sleep out his remaining days. At least when he's sleeping he's not anxious. But if he is to be a member of a normal household, without taxing it to the breaking point, he needs to maintain a reasonable schedule.

Creating just the right activity for David is difficult, because his mental, physical, and emotional capacities are now dramatically limited.

Singing in the car is one answer. The car is snug and familiar, singing old songs is calming and fun, and the action of driving lends importance to the day—even if we never reach a destination. In fact, having no destination is preferable. If we leave the car, we must redefine our context—confront the fearsome unknown. Better to stay in the car and continue singing.

In college, David was known for his fine singing voice and played numerous roles in musical productions at the University of Michigan. Later, he was the first person to sing on "live radio" in Detroit, Michigan. Even now his tenor voice is strong and melodious.

So we ride in the car, singing full-out, auditioning for Broadway, accompanied by screechy, tinny old cassettes of David's favorite musicals: *My Fair Lady, South Pacific, Fiddler on the Roof, Oklahoma, The King and I, Carousel, Music Man* ...

We harmonize and ham it up—glad there is no audience to judge us harshly. Fellow motorists look at us quizzically, but we keep our windows up and never subject them to our joyful noise.

David often speculates, "If we ever make a record, you know how many we'll sell? Two—one to me, one to you!"

Our route is not important, although we gravitate to the downtown streets. We start at Union Station, snaking our way back and forth between Eighteenth and Fourteenth all the way up to Broadway. David never tires of seeing the familiar landmarks, the expansion, the hustling city. Best of all, we're movin'!

Stalling

One way David demonstrates his anxiousness over leaving home is to stall. We have our coats on and are moving toward the door. Time and David stand still.

With his head down and one hand raised, he directs, "Wait a minute, wait … a … minute! Not so fast! What's your hurry? I need a handkerchief," or "Where in the hell did I put my glasses?" or "I'd better go to the john." He may have used the bathroom moments ago. Then he thinks of Terry: "I need to tell Terry we're leaving." Two minutes ago he kissed her good-bye. She has gone upstairs. And there is always "I need to go up and get more money." Going up to get more money can easily digress to "Speaking of money, have you seen my checkbook? It's been missing for days. Where is that sheet the bank sends me? My finances are in terrible shape. Before we do *anything*, we need to talk about my bank account."

DAVID HASN'T MANAGED his checkbook for years. Yet even though his chronology is distorted, his sense that the flow of his life has been disrupted is accurate.

If David were totally sentient, any of these detours would take a great deal of time—his gait is now so slow and unsteady. Add the scattering ash of his memory, and we slide toward infinity.

When we are free from time constraints, I accommodate several minutes of David's stalling. When a deadline is bearing down on us, I firmly thwart his every ploy. My arm in his, I propel him toward the car. His yammering persists. We address it on the fly.

I don't believe that David is afraid in a paranoid sort of way—as if something is out to get him. I believe he fears being separated from the familiar surroundings that confirm his identity.

WE HAVE JUST completed a particularly frustrating round of stalling. Finally we are at the car. Our lunch reservation is in five minutes, and the restaurant is ten minutes away. David stops again.

He looks me in the eye and says, "You know, I don't look my age, and it is a terrible disadvantage. If people knew how old I really am they would make allowances for me. As it is, they just look at me and wonder why I'm so dumb."

Suddenly the pressure to make our reservation evaporates, and my heart melts as I am drawn into David's torment. It is no longer David versus Marilyn—the tug between us as I try to move him along.

"David, it's true you don't look your age, but most people don't consider that to be a disadvantage. And I for one certainly don't think you're dumb. If I've been impatient with you, David, or have made you feel that I think you're dumb, please forgive me."

"All right, Darling. Where are we going? Aren't we in a hurry?"

DAVID ACCURATELY SENSES the discomfort of others, but he mistakenly attributes their attitude toward him to the disparity between his looks and his age. He fails to recognize that there are obstacles to interacting with him apart from his appearance or his age.

7

Facing the Inevitable

On the Waiting List

Terry, the children, and I have known for some time that David's moving to a professional care facility is inevitable. For months his name has been on the waiting list at a well-respected facility. The call has come; there is an opening. Neither David nor I have seen the place, so Terry, David, and I go for a visit.

The building is impressive. What I see inside leaves me shaken. The atmosphere is cold, sterile, fluorescent-lit. We don't see a single ambulatory resident—all are either in beds or wheelchairs. Most of those in wheelchairs are slumped and uncomprehending in front of a TV. They look tranquilized to me.

David comments, "I could never live in a place like this. Everyone here is old." He does not understand that we are visiting this place on his behalf. He is just innocently commenting.

On the side, I ask our guide if there is a wing where people are more alert and active. She says, "No, this is typical of our population."

I feel sick. David will despair and quickly deteriorate in this environment.

Renewing the Search

Back home, Terry and I prepare lunch together and discuss what we have seen. I am outspoken in my opinion.

"David will be devastated to be left among people with so little consciousness."

Terry says, "I don't have what it takes to find another place."

"I do," I reply.

"Great!" Terry says. "When will you start looking?"

"After lunch."

That afternoon, I learn a great deal and find a number of places where I *don't* want David to live. I begin to compile criteria for what I believe will be an acceptable facility. (See Appendix B: Finding the Right Home)

Masking

While researching nursing home possibilities for David, I meet one facility administrator who introduces me to the term "masking." Though I have regularly observed masking behavior in David, I learn that masking is a recognized behavior pattern commonly seen among dementia patients.

Masking is a form of bluffing, an individual's extreme effort to appear competent—a deception born of the fear of being exposed as deficient. The woman who took the time to educate me about masking also explained that it has been widely observed that an individual's masking behavior often lessens significantly in a nursing home. The belief is that, in the world at large, a person affected by dementia constantly struggles to avoid being "found out." In a nursing home, he or she realizes on some level that other residents have similar deficits. The need to maintain a facade decreases.

Once I am aware of the masking concept, I begin to recall some of David's patterns that may indicate he is struggling to save face. I have noticed that frequently he will respond to a confusing situation with "Oh, oh, oh, oh … oh, oh … oh!" David actually uses seven "ohs." I've counted them. It may take him awhile to string them together, but sooner or later he manages to work in all seven. Seven "ohs" seem to translate to "Finally! I see! I get it!" Maybe he gets it, maybe he doesn't.

Now I wonder if David's multiple "ohs" are masking. It is impossible to know, because thirty seconds after the "ohs" that seem to confirm his comprehension, David will ask the very question the "ohs" indicated he understood. Then I wonder: *Did he understand and just forget after thirty seconds that he understood, or did he pretend to understand, then forgot to hold the mask in place?*

Too frequently I catch myself obsessing over these unanswerable twists, but it is helpful to know that habitual masking is a characteristic of dementia. And masking may explain some of David's frustrating behaviors—those times when his words claim understanding but his actions demonstrate otherwise.

But I have no way of knowing for sure whether David regularly masks for me. I hope he doesn't feel the need to. One of David's frequent responses to me may be an indicator that he doesn't habitually mask for me. David often makes bold and incongruous statements that I know are incorrect, such as, "The stock market lost 500 points yesterday."

Rather than contradict him, I respond with, "I'm not aware of that David."

Invariably he answers, "Darling, don't believe a word I say unless someone else can confirm it for you. I mostly don't know what I'm talking about." This response seems straightforward and nondefensive—not typical of one who is trying to mask. Or perhaps my non-threatening response to his stock market statement allows David to *unmask* himself.

HOWEVER, just being aware that David may use masking in an attempt to preserve his self-esteem gives me another window to his reality and opens my heart wider to him. I can only imagine the torment of constantly feeling the need to disguise myself. Allowing myself to slip into a frame of mind that David might experience, I have a sense of anxiety, even panic: *I am the only one who doesn't understand—any minute I may be exposed as an imposter. I feel guilt because I am being deceptive. My guilt turns to self-loathing, because I value integrity, yet I am being deceitful—an agonizing irony, since my original intent was to preserve my self-esteem.*

We all mask to some degree. Naturally, we want to appear as smart as possible, and sometimes find that we need to camouflage, however slightly or unconsciously, the gaps in our knowledge or understanding. But for those living the nightmare of dementia, masking is a dominant and energy-sapping behavior pattern.

After I learn about masking, David and I discuss the concept. He seems intrigued that he is not alone, that dementia is widespread. There is a name for his condition and a name for the coping mechanism he uses. He expresses relief that I am aware of how hard he tries to make himself appear normal. Maybe in a nursing home David will feel less need to mask and his torment will be eased.

Postponement

Terry has gained enthusiasm for my commitment to finding just the right home for David. One morning she joins me to visit yet another place. This facility is glamorous, impressive, but not equipped to serve dementia residents.

We are referred to an affiliate residence that has not opened for business. There are no residents and no staff to observe in action—just a beautiful, untarnished shell. Not good enough. But the administrative person we speak with says all the right things. Terry is enthused. The next day, without my knowing, she puts down a deposit.

Within a couple of days the newly hired director visits David for a home evaluation. This woman is from the pat-'em-on-the-head, chuck-'em-under-the-chin school. When interacting with David she tries to compensate for his seeming lack of comprehension by raising her voice. When she talks to Terry or me, she speaks normally. Terry and I both volunteer that David has no difficulty hearing. She nods knowingly and continues to blare at him. At one point, in a singsong voice, sweet enough to gag a honeybee, she coos to him, "God didn't bless me with children, David, but he *did* give me the gift of spending my days with *special* people like you!"

With the deposit paid and the paperwork filled out, this home evaluation is the last piece of the puzzle before David can be admitted. Passionately, I argue against putting him in this facility. But Terry is finished. Soon I will come to understand how drained she really is.

It is March, and the retirement home is due to open on April 1. This date slips, slips again, then again.

Terry Is in Jeopardy

Several months prior to the decision to find a retirement facility for David, Terry has decided to give up her annual greenhouse work. Instead she has planned a two-week trip to Italy for mid-May. I am scheduled to stay with David while Terry is away.

In late April, still uncertain about David's moving date, Terry begins to experience persistent, dull headaches and dizziness. Tests show that she has temporal arteritis, a condition that, if untreated, leads rapidly to blindness. She cancels her trip and begins a regimen of Prednisone that will soon ravage her body.

Pressure is mounting. Terry is experiencing anxiety over her sudden decline. The drugs she is taking are causing profound side effects. For eight years she has watched in helpless horror as her partner has mentally evaporated. Terry is physically and emotionally exhausted. And now she faces the pain and guilt of separating from her spouse of more than six decades.

I speak with David and Terry's daughter, Sissy, in New York. In the space of a few hours we decide that David will live with me until he can settle permanently.

8

David, My Houseguest

Leaving Home

Urgently needing to relieve the pressure on Terry, we take no time to strategize. Hurriedly, Terry and I pull things from drawers and closets. David doesn't fully grasp what is happening, but he is apprehensive as he observes the preparations and resistant when we are ready to leave.

As we back down his driveway, he is finally angry and turns his fury on me: "Who do you think you are? What right do you have? Wait until my son hears about this! You'll regret this! You are out of your mind! Don't expect the slightest bit of cooperation from me! This is kidnapping! You'll never get away with this!"

What little I say is sympathetic and supportive, but anything from me incites David further. I let him vent his rage. As in the past when Terry has traveled, I cling to the hope that the passage of twelve hours will find us on higher ground. The first three hours are the worst. Miraculously, by nightfall I am no longer the enemy.

Making Adjustments

Until now, no matter how stressful my dealings with David have been, I have had the comfort of knowing I will soon be going home. Now there is no retreat. Many times a day, I must remind myself: *Breathe and focus on this one moment. You can't go home, and the cavalry's not comin'.*

The looping dialogue is interminable, and David is far more anxious and belligerent in my home than in his. Endlessly, he asks about

81

Terry and wants to know if he can call or visit her. I am feeling protective of Terry. Even without the physical challenges she is facing, she is exhausted and in a state of burnout from having been responsible for David for so long. I tell her she can call us at any time, but we will not routinely disturb her.

Being abruptly cut off from Terry is hard on David, and further convinces him that I am trying to separate him from his family. He speaks by phone with his children, but this soothes him only momentarily. He forgets he has spoken with them. There are still moments when he is convinced that I have abducted him and no one knows where he is.

Within twenty-four hours of his arrival in my home, I am on the phone with David's friends and family, instigating a card-writing campaign. Everyone rallies. Almost immediately, mail addressed to David begins to arrive—a balm more effective for him than phone calls, because mail is tangible. Perpetually he reads his cards, comforted that people know where he is and care enough about him to stay in touch.

Occasionally some of his friends call, and it is a joy to nonchalantly say, "David, it's for you." Because he forgets the calls, I start a phone call log for him—one more reminder that he has not been abandoned. Slowly, David begins to trust again that I am telling the truth. His son visits on weekends; his friends visit periodically; some even join us for lunch.

My dog and three cats provide invaluable distraction for David during our first difficult days of adjustment. Having seen him come and go in recent months, the animals are more familiar with him than he is with them. They approach him fearlessly and entertain him with their guileless antics. He is amused and flattered by their attention.

In my home the animals reign. David is accepting of this fact and even tolerant of cats on the table. He often says, "I've never liked cats, but these little dogs are different."

David does not merely tolerate the cats. He engages them and often calls my attention to them. At the breakfast table one morning, in mock alarm, he gestures accusingly toward Obi, my white Persian cat, stretched out on the newspaper that David is trying to "read." "There's a tuft of white hair on my writing table!" he offers dryly.

Obi has a soda-straw fetish. He is in a state of delirium three times a day with the appearance of a straw in David's cup. Mealtime finds Obi sitting on the table within inches of David, stalking the straw. A friendly competition evolves. Man and beast are fairly matched. They play by one rule: anything goes. Each wins often enough to keep the game alive, and the rivalry continues through David's last breakfast with us.

The dish of cat kibble is up on a counter out of the dog's reach. Frequently I find David nibbling out of this dish as if the kibble were peanuts. I remind him that he is eating the cats' food. He thinks this is a great joke. When the situation is reversed and he finds the cats eating out of this same dish—their dish—he frantically points and cries out incoherently, "The the the the ... my food ... the ... eating my food." He needs at least fifteen minutes to regain his equilibrium after one of these episodes of intense distress.

Considering the recent upheaval in David's life—leaving Terry and his own familiar surroundings, integrating into the unfamiliar environment and rhythm of my household, and adjusting to my menagerie—David is coping remarkably well.

David Runs Away

The spring weather is spectacular, and I am eager to begin refurbishing my garden. On the morning of David's third day with me, he agrees to sit at the umbrella table in the garden and talk with me while I work. We visit for a few minutes, but soon he falls asleep. As I plant, I'm feeling a sense of relief, thinking: *Despite our rocky start, this arrangement is going to work.* Noticing the slow rhythm of my breath as I take in the spring-sweet air, I feel a sense of tranquillity that has been absent for too long.

We've been in the garden for twenty minutes. Abruptly, David awakens and sulks, "Well, since nobody is paying any attention to me, I guess I'll go back inside."

"Oh, David! I'm so sorry. I thought you were dozing!"

"Yes, I bet you did. You were rude, and there is nothing else to call it. I'm going inside."

I decide there is no harm in David's going inside by himself. I'll put my tools away, rinse the dirt from my hands, and follow right behind. He huffs toward the back door, and I begin to clean up. Within five minutes I am inside. David is gone. I spend at least two minutes calling and searching each room on the four levels of the house. David is definitely gone.

I blaze out the front door. My mind is tumbling as I try to decide which way I'll turn when I reach the sidewalk. I think *left, in the direction of the busy street a block away.* But reaching the sidewalk, I look left. Nothing! I look to the right in time to glimpse David's sweater as he disappears around the corner.

Suddenly I am aware of how close I came to losing David. Had I stayed even two seconds longer in the house, I would have missed seeing him turn. We could have wandered indefinitely, not far apart, but just missing each other. I am weak, trembling, and there is an ache around what feels like a growing hollowness in my chest.

But the drama isn't over. I streak toward the corner, hoping David doesn't step in front of an oncoming car or turn another corner and disappear before I reach him. I overtake him easily, but now I have another problem: David is so agitated he refuses to return to the house with me. "I'm fed up with you—the way you treat me," he snarls. "I'm going home. I'm finished with you."

For the next ten minutes we stand on the sidewalk. David, more combative than I have ever seen him, won't even allow me to touch his arm. He demeans me as viciously as he can without resorting to obscenities.

Struggling to control my emotions, I say, "David, I would never deliberately do anything to hurt you. If my behavior was rude or thoughtless, it was unintentional. We've been friends for too long to let a misunderstanding like this damage our relationship."

Surely by now David has no idea what offense I have committed or to what behavior I am referring. Trying for a broader perspective, I begin to see him as a refugee—torn from his familiar life, thrust into a foreign land. He has neither the reference points nor the mental and emotional resources for bringing order to his chaos.

I remind myself that I am not dealing with a child. I have no lessons to teach—no fear of setting a bad precedent with an imperfect resolution. My only goal is to take David home.

Unexpectedly I hear my father's words, "The fox won't bite you because he's bad. He'll bite you because he's afraid." David is afraid. I am afraid.

"David, I'm thinking that maybe you're afraid: afraid of being in a strange place, afraid of not knowing how to return to your home, afraid that you are losing control of your life," I volunteer.

David nods. He replies, simply, "Yes."

"Well, David, I'm afraid too: afraid of your anger, afraid that I won't be able to take the best care of you when you're angry with me. I have never taken care of a ninety-three-year-old man in my home before. Sometimes I am afraid that I can't do it alone."

David, more relaxed now, takes a few moments to consider what I've said. Finally he asks, "Well, what should we do?"

"We should go back home and eat a good lunch," I respond.

He looks at me. I sense no hostility, only uncertainty. Cautiously, I take his hand. He doesn't resist. We turn to go home.

I help David into a chair at the dining room table and offer him his family photo album. Animated and content, he begins leafing through the pages.

"David, if you're comfortable looking at your album for a few minutes, I'm going to fix our lunch," I suggest.

"Sounds like a good idea, Dear! I could look at this book all day. I'm hungry too—glad you're planning to feed me!" he laughs.

David sits fifteen feet from where I'm working in the kitchen. He comments casually on his album. Several times he asks me to "come take a look" at special pictures—pictures I can describe in detail from memory.

Lost Keys

My security doors allow me to lock from the inside. Deadbolts in place, I attach the keys to my belt. Something else to add to my brochure: "Warden."

Mostly good-naturedly, David harasses me about locking him in the house and holding him prisoner.

"David, you have a condition called dementia that has caused you to lose a lot of your memory. If you walk out the door by yourself, you might not be able to find your way home. You count on me to protect you, so I keep the doors locked. But any time you want to go out, you may. We'll go together. This plan doesn't allow you to be away from *me*, and this has its disadvantages. Still, it's probably better than a poke in the eye with a sharp stick."

"Well, I don't know about that," he laughs. "I've always enjoyed the sharp stick."

ONE AFTERNOON I decide to try another quick gardening project. In fifteen minutes I plant a few containers of groundcover in a bed at the side of the house. Eight feet away on the porch, David sits supervising my work. Project complete, we go inside. When I go to lock the door from the inside, the keys are missing. This is perplexing. I had the keys recently enough to *unlock* the door when we went outside.

I return to where I was planting and filter through the mulch. Nothing. For the next several hours, I am all over the house looking for the keys. I do have a spare set, so we are not stranded, but lost keys make me uneasy. Resigned to the loss, I begin preparing our dinner.

After dinner, while cleaning up the kitchen, I flip the switch to the garbage disposal. A clanging din. The keys! Other than a few nicks, the keys are unscathed.

How did the keys come to be in the disposal? I wonder if this is David's way of retaliating for the lockdown? But even if he's the culprit, he has forgotten by now.

Active and Happy

By the end of the first week at my house, David has mellowed. We begin to expand our horizons. The grocery store, the drugstore, and the library are destinations that lure us from home. Even at this stage of dementia, David longs for activity and stimulation. However, he often likes the idea of activity more than he likes the activity itself. Inventing just the right diversion is challenging.

David was once an accomplished photographer, and I think it might be fun to buy a disposable camera for him. He is intrigued by the concept of such a camera. Once he has it, though, he seems confused and bored with the project.

He hands the camera to me. "Here, if you want pictures, take them yourself."

"Let's take turns, David. I'll go first."

"Well, alright," he agrees halfheartedly.

After several rounds of this, he warms to the activity. He begins to plan his shots. Soon he is coaching me on mine.

We finish the roll in one session. The drugstore, several blocks away, offers one-hour processing. There is scant hope that one hour from now David will remember taking the pictures. Still, I like the continuity that quick processing adds to the activity.

Once we have our pictures, David eagerly shoulders in to have a look. I remind him that he has taken most of these pictures himself. He is surprised but pleased. An astute critic, he comments on framing, lighting, and distance. Sorry that the pictures are only of the garden and the dog, he wishes we had some interesting people as subjects.

Without suggestion from me, David begins to segregate the pictures into "keepers" and "tossers."

"Hey, David, we should send some of the 'keepers' to your daughter, Sissy, in New York!"

"Good idea!" Then he reconsiders. "No, I don't know how to do that."

"That's no problem. I have Sissy's address, an envelope, and stamps. Let's put a packet together right now and take it to the post office. You can even dictate a note to include."

With real enthusiasm from David, we accomplish our mission and make it to the post office for the 5:30 pickup.

For a slow starter, the afternoon is a huge success. We've ordered a double set of prints—a good investment. This tangible component of our activity is a major benefit. David spends several hours over the next few days shuffling pictures between the "keepers" and "tossers." He also enjoys showing the pictures to his son Michael and various friends who drop by. While singing in the car is relaxing and enjoyable, a picture-taking activity, with its material reminders, can occupy David long after the pictures are taken.

DAVID LIKES TO THINK OF himself as the tireless reader he once was, but his attempts to read always fizzle. I wonder if picture books from the library would interest him, but a lengthy session at the library is not realistic for us.

I call the neighborhood library and explain to the librarian what I'm looking for and why I can't come in to browse for myself. I give her several categories that will appeal to David. She is gung-ho.

Now we have someplace to go! Several hours later we both go in to meet Amy, our book angel. She has assembled the perfect collection: eight outstanding books that will hold David's attention every day for the next three weeks.

At home, David chooses two books, and I put the rest away. I intend to rotate the books—bring out new ones as he tires of the old.

David's favorite book is *The Family of Man,* an international collection of 503 photographs that celebrates the oneness of humanity. The collection was first exhibited in the early 1950s at the Museum of Modern Art in New York. In our three remaining weeks together,

I introduce other books, but I never rotate this book out to substitute a new one. David doesn't tire of looking at these pictures and discussing them with me. If I haven't left the book by his place at the breakfast table, he asks for it, not by name but by describing it to me. "Where is that terrific book, Dear—the one with the pictures you took of all of those people?"

MOST EVENINGS AS I prepare dinner, David sits nearby looking at a book. One book is a collection of antique, theatrical advertisements dating back to Shakespeare's time. David is exuberant in his enthusiasm for these posters. Nearly every time he turns a page, he urges me to "come have a look."

One evening I give up on dinner preparations for two minutes, cut strips of sticky notes, put them into a dish, and offer them to David as bookmarks. "David, it would help me if you could mark the pages of the pictures that you want to show me. When dinner is ready, we'll sit right next to each other, and you can show me all the pictures you've marked."

Pleased to have an assignment, he marks almost every page and announces every marker. "Oh boy! Wait 'til you see this one!" "You'll be glad I saved this one for you!" "Ha! This one tops them all!"

We have a great time looking at the book together during dinner. David's analytical comments are bright and insightful: "I'm amazed at the sophistication of their marketing back then," or "The design of this one is simple, but look at how effectively they used color."

David's bookmarking and dinnertime sharing become an evening ritual. Following him on a book tour is thoroughly engaging—a great alternative to looping. He also enjoys his leadership role. And looking repeatedly at the same book with David is never boring. He brings a fresh perspective to each viewing, noticing something new every time he shares it.

DEPENDING ON THE DAY, word games are fun for us. David is sharper on some days than on others. Using elementary words, we name antonyms and synonyms. I think of familiar sayings such as "Early to bed, early to _____, makes a man _____, _____, and _____." David fills in the blanks. We talk about how the quote or proverb may have originated and perhaps the meaning of a saying like "A stitch in time saves nine."

I buy a beginner's crossword puzzle book based on historic events, and David is surprisingly knowledgeable. These activities help us pass the time, and also allow David to feel competent. If I see we have moved into an area where he is coming up with few reasonable answers, I return to a level that allows him more success.

MY CONSTANT CHALLENGE is to maintain a picture of David as a capable adult when so much of his behavior contradicts this view. It would be simpler to treat him, across the board, as a child rather than perpetually trying to determine how much of his adult self he has brought to any given moment. But the more confidence I place in David's remaining capacities, the more opportunity he has to astonish me with the depth and breadth of what he still possesses. David often astonishes me.

The Marley Snafu

After dinner one evening, I suggest that we drive to the library to drop off some books. David is eager.

My aging standard poodle, Marley, hasn't been out for a ride since David came to stay with us. I start to put a leash on Marley, but David objects, "You're not taking him along, are you?"

"Yes, I want to. Marley needs to get out as much as we do, David."

"Well, if you're taking him, I'm not going. He's a damned nuisance!"

This surprises me. David, a dog lover, has always felt a special affection for Marley, because, years ago, he had two standard poodles of his own. He often proudly points out that Marley sleeps loyally on the hardwood floor by his chair. Normally Marley would prefer to cushion his old bones on the sofa.

I can't understand David's attitude, but we'll only be gone for ten minutes, and I'm not up for a debate. I tell Marley he'll have to stay. His tail falls as David and I walk out the door.

At the library, David waits in the car while I walk the dozen steps to the book drop.

Back in the car I hear the familiar, "Now where are we going?"

"We're going home."

"Whaaaat? Already?" David objects.

"Well, we can drive downtown to see what's happening on a beautiful spring evening in the city," I offer.

"Let's go!" he says with enthusiasm.

"I'm up for it, David, but first I want to go back to the house to pick up my dog, Marley. He would enjoy a ride too."

"Fine, let's do it!" he says, reversing his earlier objection to Marley's company.

David waits in the car while I run in for Marley. I snap on the leash, and we're out the door. As Marley and I step off of my front porch and start down the path to the sidewalk, I notice that my neighbor two doors down is working in her yard. Her two dogs, a German shepherd and a husky mix, are lying on the lawn watching her.

With no provocation but with startling speed, the two unleashed dogs come howling toward us. They knock Marley to the ground and begin tearing at him. Marley is injured and screaming. I flail at the dogs. The neighbor rushes up, pulls her dogs off, and drags them home. Marley lies whimpering and bleeding. I help him to his feet. There is a large puddle of blood on the ground. I half-carry Marley back into the house, leaving a dense trail of blood all the way.

I am concerned about David, still waiting in the car. I can see him through the living room window so I know he's safe. I hope he is dozing. If I leave Marley long enough to bring David inside, Marley will wander and track blood all over the house.

Drenching a rag with cold water, I quickly wash Marley and determine that his wounds, though bleeding profusely at first, are superficial.

He is still shaking. A ride is not what he needs. Leaving him alone is not acceptable either. But David is waiting, so we venture out again.

Stepping from the evening shadows, my neighbor apologizes and offers to hose the blood from my front porch and walkway.

"Thanks, that will be helpful. Right now I need to hurry to be with my elderly friend who has been waiting for me in the car."

Ten minutes after it began, the crisis is over. Another looms inside the car. I help Marley into the backseat and settle myself behind the wheel. I heave a huge, tension-dispelling sigh and drive away.

David is silent, staring straight ahead.

"David, did you see what just happened?" I ask.

"Don't talk to me!" he responds heatedly. "You're trying to kill me! You left me alone in this car for more than two hours! Take me home immediately!" he demands.

I try to explain what happened with Marley, but David shouts me down with "You're lying! Take me home! Take me home, *now!*"

"David, you can't go home. Terry isn't well. She can't take care of you, so you're staying temporarily with me."

"Then take me to a hotel!" he insists.

"David, you can't stay by yourself in a hotel. You'd have no way to find food; you'd be lonely and frightened; you might even become lost."

"Stop this minute! Where are you taking me?" he wails.

A trip downtown is out of the question, so I am turning to go back home. "David, we're on our way home," I say quietly.

"I don't believe you. Don't try to trick me!"

We park in front of the house, and David continues his harangue, refusing to go inside.

"Michael will have plenty to say about this. Let me call Michael immediately!" he demands.

Hoping to use the phone call as a bridge from the car to the house, I tell David that we will have to go inside to make the call. His rage escalates. Pounding on the dashboard he yells frantically, "You're lying! Take me to a pay phone. You're trying to kill me!"

"David, I won't harm you in any way, but if you believe I mean to hurt you, I can understand why you're afraid."

On my cell phone, I call Michael. With David sitting beside me, I explain that I had to leave him alone in the car for ten minutes, because Marley had an accident. I tell him that David is upset and wants to talk with him. David and Michael visit briefly. David is only somewhat reassured by their conversation. He is still unwilling to go inside.

"Let's just stay here in the car for a while, David. I understand that you are very upset."

By now the sun has set. We sit silently in the darkness. David has spent his fury, but he is not budging. It's almost 8:30. I recline my seat, close my eyes, and rest. With Marley sleeping in the backseat, I am content to wait. Time is on my side.

At 9:20 David finally says, "Why the hell are we sitting here in the dark?"

"We've just been waiting until you feel ready to go into the house, David," I reply offhandedly.

"Well, I'm *ready!*" he says forcefully.

"Great! Let's go," I respond, moving swiftly before he changes his mind. What began as a simple book drop two hours ago has turned into a small nightmare. And once inside the house, David has moments of wariness. He refuses to change into his nightshirt, preferring to sleep in his clothes.

"I know you're going to try to kill me in the night. If I'm in my nightshirt, I won't stand a chance of escaping. If I'm dressed, I can run outside to call for help," he reasons.

"David, sleeping in your clothes is a fine idea, if it will make you more comfortable. And you can rest easily, David. You will be safe while you sleep," I assure him.

David won't let me approach his bed. I watch from a distance as he struggles with his blankets. Finally he is under the covers, and I turn off the lights and leave the room.

During the night, I hear David downstairs. I go down to make sure he is all right and find him standing in the middle of his room, confused.

"What time is it, Dear?" he asks.

"It's 2:10 A.M., David," I answer.

"Is it day or night?"

"It's the middle of the night," I reply.

"Well, why the hell am I dressed?" he asks, looking down at his rumpled clothes.

"Earlier you felt you would be more comfortable sleeping in your clothes. If you'd prefer to be in your nightshirt now, I can help you with it."

In his nightshirt at last, David uses the bathroom, and I help him into bed. I sit with him for a few minutes of closeness, then kiss him good night. It is 2:40 A.M.

In the morning, David greets me: "Good morning, Dear. Am I here?"

"Yes, you are, David," I reply.

"Are you here?" he asks.

"I am *definitely* here," I answer.

"Well, where *are* we?"

Another day begins.

The Human Mirror

It has occurred to me that David's seemingly unpredictable outbursts may not be so unpredictable. I have come to believe that these dramatic episodes have nothing to do with petulance or self-centeredness; I believe these incidents are fueled by terror.

When the human mirror that reflects David to David disappears, he abruptly loses himself. He has no concept of time—ten minutes, two hours—it's all the same. I believe the length and intensity of David's emotional rampages are in direct proportion to the depth and circumstance of his terror.

David wakes in the garden, doesn't see me ten feet away, and panics. If I disappear, he disappears. But my garden "disappearance" was relatively short-lived—he must have spotted me within moments of waking. His terror didn't grow to unbearable proportions, so the time it took him to dispel his terror was relatively short. Twenty minutes after his terror began, David was sitting in the dining room, looking at his photo album.

Alone in the car, waiting for me to return with Marley, David looks out the window. He sees an unfamiliar neighborhood. He doesn't remember that I have gone to get Marley so we can go for a ride. He has no context for his existence—no sense of who he is. He sees the daylight fading. His mind turns minutes to hours. The depth of his despair becomes so intense that he begins to believe he will die … alone in the darkness, lost in a strange place.

David's human mirror reappears, and he is relieved. Yet the terror that has consumed him must be dispelled. What was terror a moment before evolves into anger at having been made to feel terrified, so he rages, "You're trying to kill me!"

When Terry was away and I stayed with David in his home, at least he had his familiar surroundings to anchor him to his life. Still, he was not initially confident that I could be mirror enough to sustain his existence in Terry's absence. Over a twelve-hour period he would realize that I was a reliable mirror. He could literally "live with that."

Shower Time

David is unsteady in the shower and unable to thoroughly wash himself, so I help him. For showers I always wear shorts and a T-shirt. If David slips or has a TIA, I am prepared to dive in with him. We've never had a shower crisis, but even so, by the time David is dry and dressed, I am always drenched.

"Come on in here, Big Guy. It's Show Time!" I call from the bathroom.

"Do you want me to take off my clothes?" David asks.

"You bet. While you undress, I'll adjust the water." I make the adjustment. "Okay, David, I've adjusted the water to what *I* think is the right temperature. Check to see if you agree with me before you step in."

"I guess that will do," he drones without feeling.

"Oh no, we aren't satisfied with 'that will do.' We're looking for perfection here." I say.

"Okay, then hotter," he says. I make the adjustment. "Yes!" he says. "That's good. Oh boy! Yes, that feels good."

"Great! That's what we're after," I respond. "David, stand under the shower and get your head wet. I'm going to put some shampoo into your palm so you can wash your hair."

I put the shampoo on his hand.

He questions, "What am I supposed to do with this?"

"Put your soapy hand on your head and wash your hair, David," I coax. He takes an ineffective swipe at his head.

"That's a good start, David. May I join the fun? I'd like to give you a wonderful scalp massage."

"Sure, go ahead."

David leans into my hands like a horse being curried.

"Wow, where did you learn that?" he asks appreciatively.

"I'm not sure, David. Maybe it comes from years of being a mother. Here's a washcloth. You may want to hold it over your face while I rinse your hair. When I say three, I'm going to rinse your hair with this sprayer. The water is going to run down over your face, so be prepared."

Encouraging him to participate as much as he's able, we slowly work our way down. David arches with catlike pleasure as I scrub his back.

"David, this is liquid soap. I'm putting it into your hand so you can wash your crotch."

He makes a weak, confused attempt to wash himself somewhere around his navel. Having missed its target, the soap slides off his hand and down the drain.

"David, let's try that again. I'm going to put more soap into your hand. Now, put your soapy hand 'where the sun don't shine' and scrub like you mean it! Our social reputation depends on this. We can't have you going malodorously out into the world."

Narrowing his eyes at me, David smiles his recognition and, with determination, attacks his nether regions. I help him rinse thoroughly, and the shower is finished.

David luxuriates in the invigorating, bath-towel rubdown I give him. Unfailingly he remembers to powder himself, dousing body and floor in equal measure.

AN HOUR OF OUR MORNING is gone, and we haven't eaten breakfast yet. To save time, I help David into his clothes. Although he enjoys my assistance and laughs at the idea of having his own "female valet," I avoid helping him dress on those mornings when he doesn't shower. I believe that dressing himself is an important competency for him to maintain. This is an activity he can do independently— one of the few areas of mastery left that allows him to be in charge. Dressing provides David with an opportunity for accomplishment at the beginning of every day. Each night, however, I lay out his clean clothes for the next morning. Left on his own, David will wear the same dirty clothes indefinitely.

Soon we are eating breakfast. Side by side, we leaf through the morning paper. David can no longer read an article from start to finish. There is nothing wrong with his ability to read. He simply does not retain enough information from one sentence to the next to provide the continuity necessary for understanding. Often he is perturbed because he can't comprehend what he reads. Mostly, reading the paper means commenting on the ads and repeating a headline aloud a dozen times or more, occasionally asking, "What the hell are they talking about?" Left alone at this activity, he quickly falls asleep.

"DAVID, WHILE YOU FINISH reading the paper, I'm going to take a quick shower."

"Can I help you do that? Wash your back—anything?" he asks hopefully.

"Hey, thanks for the offer, David. I've got it covered. I'll be down in fifteen minutes."

"That's not fair! You got to help *me* shower."

"That's right, David. The difference is, you needed help. I don't need help."

"But I *want* to help you," he persists.

"Not today—not any day, my friend. That's my final answer," I say as I leave the table.

I'm in the shower. I hear an urgent pounding on the bathroom door.

"David, is that you? What do you need?"

"I want to wash your back!" he yells.

"Thanks anyway, David. I don't need your help."

The pounding becomes louder and more urgent. When I don't respond, he works the doorknob rhythmically, then begins to rapidly jerk the locked door back and forth in the jamb.

"David, stop that pounding immediately! I deserve some peace while I shower!" The onslaught ceases.

Soon I hear the drawers of my bedroom dresser opening and closing. In one sweep I am out of the shower, throwing on my robe, and opening the bathroom door. Across the hall, in my bedroom, David is rummaging through my lingerie drawer. I am looking at him in profile. He is bent over. With revulsion I realize that his mouth is open, and long viscous strands of drool are dripping onto my lingerie.

"David! Please, leave my bedroom right now! You are a guest in my home. My bedroom is off limits to you! You need to finish reading your newspaper. I'll join you downstairs in a few minutes."

I am surprised when David abruptly leaves my room, without protest, and goes downstairs. Feeling invaded, disheartened, I return to my shower.

Later in the day, I find David sifting through a filing cabinet in my office. Again I explain that he is a guest in my home, and it is rude for him to rifle through my belongings. He sees the situation from a "mi casa es su casa" perspective and is insulted at the suggestion of boundaries.

LIVING WITH DAVID is so challenging. I need a refuge. Until now the upper level of the house—my bedroom, office, and bathroom—has been my sanctuary. Now I realize I have no haven. Having watched David stir through my personal belongings, I know that no amount of intellectualizing, like: *When I am out of his sight, David probably just needs to look for clues to his own identity*, is going to help me feel less invaded.

Finally I am beginning to fully appreciate why people who care for those who have dementia need regular time away and a physical space that is theirs alone. I could never quite understand why Terry was adamant about David's using his own bathroom and not hers. Now I know.

The Lamp Fiasco

David is in his nightshirt. As soon as he brushes his teeth, washes his face, and uses the toilet, he'll be ready for bed. I outline his three-point agenda and tell him that I am going to the laundry room to start a load of his dirty clothes. The laundry room is six steps down from where we are standing. I leave him in the bathroom, his loaded toothbrush in his hand, his washcloth on the edge of the sink.

The dirty clothes are already piled at the top of the stairs. Scooping them up, I hurry to the washing machine. In record time I turn to go back to David. I've been away from him no more than two minutes.

Thud! Crash! Shattering glass! I bolt up the stairs. David is collapsed in a corner, behind the sofa, wrapped around my much-cherished, and now-demolished, antique torchère floor lamp.

Curious, the animals are circling, padding through the shards of glass that have sprayed out in an immense radius.

David is moaning, "Ohhh! Ohhh! Ohhh!"

"David, are you okay?" I ask, knowing that my words express concern but my tone conveys frustration.

"Oh! … Yes! … That takes the wind out of a guy! … A big surprise!"

"Well, I'm glad you're not hurt, David, but I'm furious with you! I left you in the bathroom to brush your teeth, wash your face, and use the john. You evidently didn't do *those things*, but instead came over here where you had no need to come, worked your way behind the sofa, broke my irreplaceable antique lamp, endangered my animals, and created a huge mess that will take me an hour to clean up!"

Shooing the animals out of the fray, I turn to help David to his feet.

"What did you expect me to do? I couldn't sleep with the light on! I had to pull out the plug!" is his lame and quarrelsome comeback.

"Right now I am so angry, David—I don't even want to look at you or hear your voice. Let me help you into bed, then I'll clean up this mess."

"Oh no, I can't go to bed yet, I need to help you!"

"David, you'll help me most by quickly getting into bed so you don't continue to scatter this broken glass and grind more of it into my carpet."

As I steer him toward his bed he continues, "Well, I'm not going to …"

"David, please, stop!"

"But you have to let me …"

"David, no more!"

"But I think you …"

"David! Enough!"

"Why can't I just …"

"David, you are in a *danger zone!* I can't remember when I was this angry! You will be a lot better off if you *don't say anything!*"

I help David into bed. I leave his room to get the vacuum and a cardboard box for the larger pieces of glass, saying over my shoulder as I go, "Don't get out of bed, David. You will only make a bad situation worse. Believe me, you don't want to see me any angrier than I am right now!"

Returning, I begin the cleanup.

Wisely, David remains in bed, but he hollers out a constant prattle in competition with the vacuum's drone. I can't hear what he's saying. He chatters on, and I feel somehow soothed by the white noise of the vacuum that forms a protective barrier between us.

PART OF MY ANGER stems from the nagging suspicion that David didn't complete his bathroom tasks because he was annoyed that I had left him in favor of starting the laundry. I have a hunch that he intended to quickly turn out the lights and hurry into bed to make it seem as if I had neglected him for a long time: *Wait a minute! Is this the beginning of paranoia? Is this what happens to isolated caregivers?* I wonder.

Maybe David simply did not understand what was expected of him. Maybe he was innocently improvising—doing his best. But I am left with two certainties: I can't be sure of David's motives, and I am close to the limit of my endurance.

It seems a pattern is emerging. Too often, when David doesn't have my full attention, he becomes belligerent. I resent this, feeling at once claustrophobic, manipulated, and despairing, because I know I can't give him better care or more attention than I'm already giving him. Maybe David is just afraid of being alone and losing himself. But I feel like I'm losing *myself*—under siege, not at my charitable best.

I want to believe that my fury over the broken lamp would have been more restrained if I had not been confined with David for so long. The stress of being the sole caregiver for one who has dementia is immeasurable. Without having experienced it, no one can fully appreciate the magnitude of the demands on all levels—physical, mental, and emotional.

For years I have been with David and have cared for him during numerous five-day stints. I thought I was fully aware of his deficits and my own capacities, but I underestimated the strain of single-handedly caring for him for weeks without respite. Nothing could have prepared me for the reality of living with David, and I had no way of gauging my limits beforehand.

Occasionally I still find slivers of glass in the carpeting and furniture at the site of the lamp fiasco. Momentarily I feel nostalgic. At the time of the brouhaha, I could not have imagined that reminders of that night would inspire anything close to nostalgia.

Nocturnal Wandering

Terry has often mentioned that David awakens in the middle of the night, dresses, and rouses her to accommodate his chauffeuring or food-preparation demands.

When staying with David at his house during Terry's absences, I have also experienced his wakefulness. I sleep just down the hall from him. I awaken at the first distinctive sound of shish ... shish ... shish—his slow feet on carpet—before he has a chance to dress and come up with an agenda. I call to him. He comes into my room, I reorient him to the time, and he goes amiably back to bed. Being an easy sleeper, I return quickly to sleep. No big deal.

When David comes to live with me, my attitude changes. His nocturnal wanderings become significant. He sleeps two levels down from where I sleep. Sometimes I hear him, but usually I have no early warning that he is awake and wandering. Maybe I am too exhausted to hear him feeling his way on the dark stairs just outside my open door. He finds my bed and leans silently over me. I jerk to consciousness—see him silhouetted in the dark. My heart tries to hammer out of my chest.

IT IS AROUND 3 A.M. David, fully dressed, is indignantly demanding his breakfast—*as if I am a slacker!* I feel the necessity to go downstairs with him to help him back into bed.

In my own bed again, I'm wired—hopelessly awake. A major adrenaline zap, frustration with David, and just enough rest to take the edge off my tiredness are no sleeping tonic.

After an extended time of being David's sole caregiver, I am depleted by the time I go to bed each night. I need eight hours away from David to rejuvenate myself. I have to admit that, interrupted sleep and inconvenience aside, I resent being wakened in the middle of the night when there is no problem. No amount of intellectualizing makes me totally understanding and compassionate at 3 A.M. when I have given David my unceasing focus all day for so many days without a break.

Until now I have believed that I could pretty much go with the flow, put a philosophical spin on things, surmount the insurmountable, cope. Now I feel humbled. "Achilles' heel," "Waterloo," "nemesis," "daunted" come frequently to mind.

Never have I judged Terry harshly, but now I have tremendous empathy for her and the long road she has traveled. And I know that I can't fully understand the scope of what she has dealt with. She has the additional emotional conflict of being David's sixty-four-year marriage partner. Her ambivalence must be profound.

I myself have gained sixty-five pounds in the last year and a half. Food has been my instant and reliable solace—my reward and replenishment for the physical and emotional energy that is being vacuumed out of me. For months, I've been gravitating too frequently toward the bakery, ice cream shop, and candy store. I seem to have an insatiable need to soothe and comfort myself.

And my burden is light compared to the burden of the solitary caregiver of a family member. Excluding this time when David is living with me and the periodic five-day stints when Terry has traveled, I have never been fully responsible for his care.

Another factor with which I do not have to contend is family dynamics: the unresolved emotional issues present in *every* family that unavoidably find their way to the caregiving arena and magnify the stress.

I am coming to see that caring for one who has dementia produces crushing stress levels. Surely the stress intensifies manyfold for those who care for their life partner or other loved one. I am sobered by the thought of adding to my own experience the grief of seeing a family member's rapid decline; of adding the guilt that results from simultaneous love yet unavoidable resentment—resentment that overwhelms when a solitary caregiver has given too much care without respite; of adding what must be the supreme guilt when one makes the decision to relinquish the caregiving of a loved one to professionals in an institution.

Too Much Decaf

David's appetite for coffee is insatiable. As long as I have known him, Terry has tried to limit his coffee, even though he drinks instant decaf. I believe at age ninety-three, a guy should have whatever he wants … in whatever quantity he wants it. Wrong! I learn the hard way that large quantities of decaf cause David to have massive bouts of diarrhea that are difficult to quell.

Soon after he arrives at my house, the effects of my liberal coffee policy are evident in David's frequent and urgent trips to the bathroom.

One of David's bathroom visits results in his needing a complete change of clothes. I learn this via closed-door communication. Entering the bathroom to deliver his clean ensemble, I am dizzied by the stench. Liquid excrement has been smeared randomly on many surfaces. Further, I see that one entire shelf of the small ornamental bookcase that stands within reach of the toilet is packed with wads of diarrhea-drenched toilet tissue. Instead of flushing these, for some reason David has preserved them.

I help David into the shower for a rinse-off; I help him dress; I begin bathroom reclamation.

Later, when he is getting ready for bed, I notice a dribble of diarrhea on his slacks and toss them onto the dirty clothes pile.

"Hey! What did you do that for?" he asks indignantly.

"These are dirty, David. They have diarrhea on them," I say, showing him.

"Oh, don't be silly! That's not enough to worry about!" he argues.

"David, you have always been meticulous about your grooming. Even a speck of diarrhea on your pants is enough for a meticulous man to worry about. That's one of the reasons you have me around: to help keep you lookin' dapper. Dapper and diarrhea are incompatible!"

"Alright, Dear. You're very persuasive. I'll go along with it."

The Army

There are whole days when David is obsessed with finding a way out of the army. Then he will go for several days without mentioning the army. Just when I think the subject has been put to rest, he'll pick up the thread again and follow it back into the quagmire.

"Can you help me get out of the army, Dear? I need to write my letter of resignation, but I think I'll need your help. I'm pretty upset about this. On the one hand, I am desperate to get out. I don't think I can put up with the army another day, so I'm hoping they will accept my resignation. But I'll feel embarrassed if they just say, 'Okay.' I really want them to say, 'Gee, Dave, we understand that you want to resign, because you've put in a lot of good years. But we can't let you go. You're too valuable to the operation.' That's what I *want* them to say, but that would be hard too, because I *have to* get out!"

David has never been in the military. I wonder if his obsession with resigning from the army is symbolic of his sometimes-stated desire to resign from life.

Home to Michigan

At other times David is consumed with the idea of returning to Michigan.

"How can I get back to Michigan? Can I drive back to Michigan?"

"David, a road trip to Michigan sounds like fun, but you don't drive anymore."

"Well, let's say I *hired* a fella to drive me to Michigan."

"Even if you could find someone to drive you to Michigan, David, we have another problem: your doctor and dear friend, Abe Kauvar, has advised you not to travel. Also, it has been many years since you've been in Michigan. You left Michigan in 1937 when you were thirty-two years old. You've lived in Colorado for more than sixty years. You no longer have friends in Michigan."

"Well, you're wrong about that, but I'm not going to argue with you. The main thing is getting there. Let's say I hired a fella to drive me to Michigan …"

"But we're still overlooking the fact that Dr. Kauvar has said you *must not* travel."

"Hmmm … I guess that settles it then."

And "that" always does settle it … for a matter of minutes. But once in the back-to-Michigan groove, we are destined to dance many rounds of the Michigan Reel.

DAVID HAS LIVED IN Denver for two-thirds of his life, far longer than he lived in Michigan. His three children were born in Denver; his career flourished in Denver; he has contributed significantly to the Denver community. Yet he experiences a recurring and undeniable tug in the direction of his childhood roots. David's yearning to "go home" may not be unique. I have heard that many elderly people long to return to the place where they spent their early years. I wonder if humans have a natural desire, even an instinct, to complete their life's geographical circle—one more step toward final closure.

On the Phone with My Friend

One evening I am in the kitchen preparing dinner when my friend, Chris, calls. While talking on the phone, I continue cooking, setting the table, and making all the necessary preparations so we can eat on time. After twenty minutes I hang up.

Instantly David grouses, "Well, this is just great! You can talk for an hour on the phone, but you can't seem to find the time to fix my dinner."

"Au contraire, David, I've been cooking while I was talking. Dinner is ready. We can sit down immediately. We're having one of your favorites: shrimp-garlic sauté."

"Well, you were inconsiderate to ignore me for so long. I don't want to eat with someone who is so inconsiderate. I won't be eating dinner tonight."

"Suit yourself, David. I'm going to eat right now. If you change your mind, I'll welcome your company."

Nothing more is said, and David eats no dinner. He has no way of knowing that it is the brief and infrequent interludes on the phone with my friends, a lifeline to the outside world, that have made it possible for me to minister so long without respite to his needs.

9

Willowglen

A Home for David

Initially, I believe I have signed up for a week with David in my home. But the retirement home continues to miss target dates for opening. The "week" becomes nearly a month.

In the third week of May, I begin on my own to look for another residence for David. A close family friend of his, aware that I'm looking, calls to tell me about Willowglen. After a phone interview with Willowglen's community coordinator, I am hopeful. Terry is still too sick to participate in renewed efforts to find a home for David. She has no energy to waste on false starts, so I don't involve her prematurely. But I tell Sissy and Michael about Willowglen, and we all agree I should take David there for a visit.

At Willowglen, David and I meet the staff and the residents and have a full tour of the facility. I am impressed. David is wholeheartedly enthusiastic at each new revelation: the massage room, the Jacuzzi, the exercise room, the activity rooms, the wide-screen TV, the expansive and inviting outdoor areas. But I am certain that David is not imagining his own residency at Willowglen.

Encouraged by our visit, I call Terry to tell her what I have done. She is receptive to exploring the possibility of Willowglen. I arrange for the three of us to return for a visit the next day. Terry is satisfied and believes Willowglen is right for David. The following day, he and I return for his evaluation. Before we leave, the director signals me: He's in!

Grief and Preparation

There is so much to be done: paperwork to complete, arrangements to be made for moving furniture, and David himself will need extra support through this time of major transition in his life. Knowing that it will be impossible to predict David's capacity to comprehend and retain the information regarding his impending move, I decide to withhold nothing but to introduce the information gradually and repeatedly.

In the days before I move David to Willowglen, I experience powerful waves of melancholy. I watch my brave friend doing his confused best to cope with life in my simple household—just the two of us and my animals. For nearly a month David has been the primary focus of my attention. Even with my attentive and nurturing support, he has been stressed. I agonize over the terror he will surely feel when he is in strange surroundings with no familiar faces—when he is just one more needy person in a group of many like himself. Who will travel back to Michigan with him, applaud his life's accomplishments, recognize *him*, know *he* had a brilliant mind, realize *he* has a proud history, even when he appears to be a blank slate?

Biography

Attempting to ease David's transition and my anguish, I decide to prepare a detailed biography sheet to which he can refer and be reminded of who he is. I also want this biography sheet to be something of himself that he can share with anyone who has the time and interest in glimpsing a broader view of David Touff—the man who once was, and the man who still retains the essential characteristics of his former self.

David sits with me at the dining room table as I begin to lay out the various milestones in his life. Of course, putting all the pertinent information on paper takes longer with David present, but it is after all, his life, and writing his biography with his input, is rewarding for David and enjoyable for me. Surprisingly, he remembers details from his early years: his elementary school friend, Warner Law, his father's dry goods store business, his father's decision to move the family from Freeland, Michigan, when David reached high school age so David could receive a better education.

Over the period of several days, David and I work on the biography. I call Terry for her input and confirmation of dates. When we finish and I present him with a printed copy, David whoops, "Hey, this is me! Where did this come from?"

DAVID TOUFF

Born	August 3, 1905—Freeland, Michigan
School	Elementary—Freeland, Michigan
	High School—Northern High School— Detroit, Michigan
	College—University of Michigan— Ann Arbor, Michigan
Married	Terry Fiske—June 14, 1935
Children	Daniel Touff—Born 1941—Died 1963
	Michael Touff—Attorney—Denver
	Terry (Sissy) Cooper—Editor—New York
Grandchildren	Daniel and Katie (Michael's children)
	Joshua and Abigail (Sissy's children)
Work	1925–1937 Department Store— J. L. Hudson, Detroit
	1937–1969 Department Store— May Company, Denver
	1959–1969 President, Department Store— May D&F, Denver
	1969–1979 International Executive Service Corps—Columbia, Hong Kong, Indonesia, Iran, Mexico, Turkey (some countries twice)
Community Service	Cofounder KOA Television
	Head of Denver Planning Commission— Early 1950s

	Member of Development Group for Auraria Campus
	Established (with wife, Terry) the Touff Memorial Scholarship Fund in Chemistry Department at University of Colorado
Board of Directors	Colorado National Bank
	National Jewish Hospital
	University of Denver
	Denver Art Museum
Interests	Reading
	Writing
	Photography
	Tennis
	Ballroom Dancing
	Music—Singing Show Tunes
	Collecting Folk Art
	World Travel
Favorite Things	Animal—Dog
	Color—Blue
	Country to visit—Mexico
	Foods—Apple Pie, Bananas, Grapes, Hamburgers, and Shrimp
Favorite Memories	Growing up in Freeland, Michigan
	Marriage to Terry Touff
	Fatherhood
	World travel with Terry and children
	Many loyal dogs

Reminders

I also prepare a "reminders" sheet that will explain to David where he is, why he is there, where his family is, and his current, solid relationship with his family.

DAVID TOUFF
Denver, Colorado, U.S.A.
Reminders

- David's wife, Terry, and his two children, Michael and Sissy, love David deeply. They write to him and visit him often.
- David was 94 years old on his last birthday, August 3, 1999.
- David moved to Denver, Colorado, in 1937 to work for the May Company.
- David has lived in Denver for 63 years.
- David's wife, Terry, is 88 years old.
- David's wife, Terry, is no longer strong enough to take care of David in their home in Denver.
- David now lives permanently at Willowglen, a retirement home in Denver that specializes in caring for people who have dementia.
- Dementia is a condition with symptoms of memory loss, disorientation, loss of vocabulary, and general confusion.
- David is often confused and anxious about his situation.
- David is often frustrated, because he feels he has lost a great deal of his vocabulary.
- David often says he knows what he wants to say, but he cannot find the words to express himself.
- Willowglen, the place where David lives, is located in east Denver, about 15 minutes away from David's wife, Terry, and his son, Michael.
- David's friends and family visit David at Willowglen in Denver.
- David's family (his wife, Terry, and his two children, Michael and Sissy) have arranged for David to live at Willowglen in Denver where David will be safe and well cared for at all times.

To avoid confusing David, I prepare two reminders sheets: the first, in future tense, appropriate for our discussions leading up to David's move, for example, "David will soon live permanently at Willowglen"; the second, in present tense, appropriate after David moves to Willowglen, for example, "David now lives permanently at Willowglen."

I SEND BOTH THE biography and reminders sheets to Terry, Michael, and Sissy for their approval. I label all of the pictures in David's album so he won't be confused when he looks at them alone or embarrassed when he shows them to others and can't remember the names of his loved ones. In the front of the album I put the biography and reminders. I also frame a copy of the reminders that will stand on David's dresser at Willowglen.

The week before David moves to Willowglen, I put the reminders by his place at the table and we discuss them at every meal and in between. Truly, we talk of little else. Most of the time, David seems to comprehend and accept the picture I am painting for him of the changes he is about to experience. Repeatedly he expresses appreciation for the information.

In my bed the night before David enters Willowglen, I am restless, going over all the details of my logistical plan for the move. I am determined that the transition will be as smooth and tranquil for David as I can make it.

Contemplating what lies ahead for him, I am suddenly overcome with grief. I feel both sad and guilty, realizing that I know more about David's life than he does. But I decide that maybe this is not all bad. David, in his ignorance, is already asleep, while I, with more knowledge, lie brooding. Still, I cry myself to sleep.

Moving Day

The morning of the move, we're up early, showering, singing, and eating a good breakfast together. The day is off to a good start. But as I begin to carry his things to the car, David becomes anxious.

"Hey wait a minute, where are you going with my things?"

"Remember? We were discussing it at breakfast, David. This is moving day. You are moving to Willowglen, the retirement home, remember?"

"I don't know what the hell you're talking about. You don't have the authority to move me *anyplace!*"

"This is not my idea, David. You and your family have agreed that this move is the best thing for all of you. I'm only driving you there."

"Why didn't anyone tell me? This is the first I've heard of it! People don't tell me the important things anymore!"

"David, as soon as I come back inside, we'll talk more about this situation."

Between every trip I make to the car, we repeat the "Hey, wait a minute, where are you going with my things?" scenario. Finally I say, "David, I need you to help me out. Will you sit here at the table and read over this sheet and check out the photo album?"

Every time I pass through the room and hear "Hey, wait a minute," I reply, "Can't stop now, David. I'm carrying a heavy load. The answers to all of your questions are on that sheet you're holding. Be sure to start reading at the top."

The reminders save my sanity, comfort David, and allow us to arrive at Willowglen at the appointed hour. Seeing the information in writing seems to diffuse David's anxiety. When he reads the information, the move doesn't feel like something cruel that I am imposing on him. The writing gives the information an authority that is compelling. It is written. It is true.

I HAVE MADE AN appointment for David to have a haircut so he will arrive at Willowglen looking his best. This stop at a familiar place, his regular barbershop, seems to soothe him. As we continue on our way, David is serene.

Terry is waiting for us at Willowglen. David is thrilled to see her after nearly a month of separation. He sits contentedly and watches us making his bed, hanging pictures, putting his fresh towels in the bathroom. David's son Michael stops by to say hello and this further buoys David's spirits. I'm certain he doesn't suspect that soon we will all be leaving him.

The actual moment of parting is not dramatic. Terry leaves. A staff member joins David and me. I move toward the door, saying goodbye. There is a final "Hey, wait a minute ..." I remind David that he will be staying at Willowglen. I hold his face between my hands, kiss him, hug him, and tell him I love him. "I'll see you tomorrow, David," I offer as I slip out the door into the late afternoon sun. I am numb. I don't cry.

AFTER SIX MONTHS OF living at Willowglen, David always greets me with "Where in the hell did you come from, Darling?" Then he points to the framed "Reminders" on his dresser. "Take a good look at that," he says. "Best thing in this room. I read it ten times a day." With a black permanent marker, he has marked on the glass the lines he considers to be most important—the lines that define his condition and his relationship to his family.

10

Living at Willowglen

First Days

David's first days at Willowglen are anxious ones. He experiences
many of the same emotions he had when he came to live with me.
Again the realization that he cannot come and go at will is sobering.

THE MORNING WE LEAVE for Willowglen, David has about $90 in
his billfold. I wonder if this money will be secure. In the end I make
the conscious choice to let him keep it. The possible loss of $90
seems a reasonable price for allowing him the dignity of keeping his
money. By the end of the second day, all but $2 of the money has dis-
appeared. David does not necessarily feel that someone has stolen his
money. He just knows he doesn't have any. Being without cash makes
him frantic. No amount of reassurance that everything is paid for
calms his anxiety. He misses the sense of security and independence
that comes from having cash in his pocket.

A STANDARD PROCEDURE AT Willowglen is to lock residents' closets. The goal is to protect each person's belongings from other residents and to prevent individuals from misplacing or damaging their
own belongings.

The locked closet is troubling to both David and me. I believe that
David needs the comfort of seeing and touching the things that are
familiar to him. To lock him out of his own closet seems demeaning
and unnecessarily harsh.

After speaking with one of David's caregivers, I alter the lock on
his closet to allow him free access. Within days he becomes obsessed

with his clothes, spreading them out on the floor and walking on them as if they're not there.

When I first question David about his behavior, he says he has too many clothes, and he is sorting out the ones he wants to give away. Later he says he is laying his clothes out for packing, because he is going home soon.

This happens repeatedly. His clothes become soiled and need to be laundered, making more work for the staff. Reluctantly, sadly, I lock his closet.

The Haircut

It is my bias that mentally impaired people are at such a formidable social disadvantage that at least their grooming should be impeccable. Few people, it appears, share this view. I have noticed, for example, that haircuts for the mentally challenged population tend to be carelessly performed, utilitarian necessities. I wonder if there is a pervasive bad-haircut conspiracy. A guy begins to lose his mental edge? Give him the bad haircut. He'll be easily spotted in a crowd. We can all glance sideways at him and contemplate his oddness. And if he is still alert enough, he can notice these sideways glances and busy himself with uneasy wondering about why people look at him furtively.

After David's first hack haircut at Willowglen, I take him to his regular barber. This marks our first outing since his move. We pass through locked doors into a world free from regimen, a world unobstructed by high walls, a world blessedly free from the formulaic, plastic perkiness of some well-meaning interior decorator whose efforts to visually euphemize the face of sadness are the more melancholy for the attempt.

"Wait! Where are we going in such a hurry?" David questions anxiously.

"You have an appointment for a haircut with Dick. Isn't it great to be out in the world on an escapade together? Just like old times, huh, David?"

"But I don't have my suitcase! We have to go back."

"David, you won't need your suitcase at the barbershop."

"How would you know what I need?"

"You're right, David, I don't always know what you need. You will be at Dick's for only twenty minutes, though. I'm guessing that you won't need your suitcase."

"Will we go directly to the airport from the barbershop, or can we pick up my suitcase after my haircut?"

"We aren't going to the airport today, David. We're on our way to Dick's barbershop."

"Well, I can tell you right now, you're going the wrong way. Hey, where are you taking me?"

"I know why you think I'm going the wrong way, David. We've never taken this route to Dick's before. We're almost there."

"How long have we lived here in New York?"

"We live in Denver, Colorado, David."

"You're wrong about that, but I don't want to argue with you."

"We have both traveled to New York many times, but neither of us has ever lived in New York. We live here … in Denver."

"We live in Denver? Well, I'll be damned! Gosh, I'm glad we're together. I'm learning things I never knew before! But are we going to miss the plane? Say! What about my suitcase?"

"Here we are, David."

"My God! This is where I get my hair cut! How in the hell did you know I was coming here? How did you find your way here?"

"I made the appointment for you, David. We've been here many times together. I know the way."

"Will you wait for me? How will I get to the airport?"

"While Dick cuts your hair, I'm going to the bank. By the time you're finished, I'll be back to take you home."

"Home? Do we have time to go home before we go to the airport?"

"I'll be back in plenty of time to pick you up, David."

After his haircut, we drive down Sixth Avenue, away from the barbershop. He sees the landmarks, familiar for so many years, and he starts to cry.

"David, do you have a problem?" I ask gently.

"*Yes,* I have a problem!" he wails. This is my home! I never see it! I'm not here! I miss this place! Wow! What a maneuver! Did I ever tell you you're a hell of a good driver, Dear?"

I HAVE DISCOVERED that with David's dementia-related torment has also come the relief of easy distraction. In the fraction of a fleeting moment, he can leap from melancholy to glee. And yes, David has always appreciated my driving. For him it's part of the adventure. "Riding with you, Darling, is the next best thing to driving myself," he frequently applauds. I suspect that my assertive (some say rowdy) style of driving allows him a vicarious pleasure—perhaps a feeling that he himself is teasing the limits.

ER at Midnight

It's 9 P.M. when the phone rings. Sarah, a nurse at Willowglen, is calling to tell me that David has a severe earache. He says he won't be able to sleep. Sarah is about to go off duty and doesn't want to leave for the night without resolving the situation. She doesn't demand that I take David to the emergency room, but she suggests that she will be more comfortable if I do.

I am scheduled to leave town early in the morning for a one-day trip. If there is ear trouble brewing for David, I want to address it before I go away.

Willowglen is thirty minutes from my home. It is after 9:30 P.M. when I arrive there. David, coat on, is waiting for me. Smiling and twinkle-eyed, he greets me as if I were a party guest. I ask him about the pain in his ear. "Pain?" he asks. "In my ear? I don't believe there is a pain in my ear, but I do have a hell of a sore throat!" I notice that he has some chest congestion. However, by the time we walk to the car, the congestion has dissipated, shaken loose by the exercise.

David is in high spirits as we venture out into the crisp October night. This is the most fun he's had in months. I am amazed at his lack of anxiety. He is repetitive and confused at times, but overall, thrilled to be on an adventure.

As we drive along, David asks, "How old am I anyway?"

"Two months ago you turned ninety-four, David,"

"Ninety-four! People aren't supposed to live to be that old … are they? This is ridiculous! How does a guy get out of here?"

"Nature takes its course, David. We don't need to do anything but enjoy the ride."

"Well, I'm certainly enjoying this ride!" he laughs. "Do you know where you're going?"

At the hospital David immediately charms the admissions nurse, and she is pleasantly responsive to his claim, "I helped build this place." But I sense her bemusement that David is in the emergency room at 10:30 at night, in good humor, with no apparent symptoms. She must wonder why I've rousted out this lovely old man for late-night, emergency-room examination.

We are ushered into our own curtained cubicle. I help David change into a gown. Of course, he is chilly, so I cast about for blankets. When, at last, David is snugly wrapped and comfortable on his gurney, he needs to use the toilet. We undo what we've just done and set out.

Back from the men's room, rebundled and on his gurney, David tries to strike up a conversation with a seemingly inebriated man who lies on another gurney just beyond the partitioning curtain. David indicates with a hand gesture that he thinks the man is cuckoo, yet he doesn't let an opportunity pass to inform the man, "You probably don't know it, but I helped build this place!" This information is evidently lost on our neighbor. No response. Perhaps he's gesturing to someone on his own side of the curtain that the man on our side is cuckoo.

Around midnight, a doctor appears for five minutes. He pronounces David's ears "clear," his chest "clear," his throat "maybe a little red." He prescribes Tylenol for any pain David might have. He also orders a rapid-strep culture. We wait twenty minutes for a nurse to arrive to do the throat swab, then another thirty minutes to receive the negative result. Hardly rapid.

On our way back to Willowglen, David complains bitterly about the pain of his sore throat. Is he wily enough to try to prolong our outing? He may be. Nevertheless, I stop at an all-night market to buy some zinc lozenges for him. He says they help.

At Willowglen, I help David into his nightshirt, wait as he executes his nighttime ablutions, and kiss him good night.

It's a few minutes after 2 A.M. when I finally lie in my own bed. Before drifting off I reflect on the five bizarre hours I have just devoted to David and on the consuming nature of caring for one who has dementia. Once again I have experienced firsthand the reality of a family's responsibility—ongoing and unpredictable.

Next morning before leaving town, I call Willowglen to check on David. He is fine—no hint of a problem.

Moving to Meadow House

When David first moves to Willowglen, I am especially attuned to him, wanting to be sure that he doesn't slip into an institutional abyss. My expectation is that he will have a challenging time of adjustment. after which he will settle in at a reasonable level of comfort. After several weeks David's initial anxiety diminishes, but I am troubled: his zest is gone.

DAVID'S CARELESS GROOMING is another red flag that lets me know we have a problem. If I see him on Tuesday and return on Thursday, he will likely be wearing the same soiled shirt and slacks. Most of the time he is unshaven; his hair is oily and disheveled.

Fastidious grooming is no longer one of David's priorities. Even so, I have always observed a marked change in his morale once he is showered, shaved, and dressed attractively. I know he will feel better and see the world differently if his grooming is at a consistently high level. Of equal concern, however, is how the *world* sees David. Now more than ever, he needs people to be close to him, and I view his careless grooming as a barrier to closeness.

Research has revealed that the brain center that serves the sense of touch is the only center not affected by the plaque and tangles of Alzheimer's disease. Even more reason to assist David toward the goal of being more touchable.

The problem is not a simple one. David has not established a close rapport with his caregivers. Most of them are from foreign countries and their accented English is difficult for him to understand. Also, he may be trying to assert his independence by resisting help when it is offered.

When I was David's caregiver, there came a time when I no longer offered grooming help, I just gave it. By that time, though, we already had a long history together. Rather than taking a good-humored but assertive approach with David, I see his caregivers being subservient toward him. He needs strong leadership and respectful care, delivered with humor. He is not receiving these.

WILLOWGLEN CONSISTS OF four "houses" that are laid out around a central common area of administrative offices and activity rooms. Each house serves thirteen residents who are assigned to a house based on space availability, not on their level of functioning. David lives in Brook House. I begin to observe that the residents and staff in Meadow House are operating on a much higher level. I want David to live in Meadow House.

Moving David will no doubt subject him to another adjustment period, but I believe the significant improvement in his environment will outweigh the short-term disruption in his life. Fortunately, there is a vacancy in Meadow House. Terry agrees to David's moving, and I begin to strategize.

The floor plans of all four houses are identical and I am hopeful that his familiarity with the layout will ease the transition. I mention the move to David. He seems indifferent to the prospect. Maybe he doesn't understand what I'm proposing. Maybe he doesn't care if he moves, because he has no attachments to either the caregivers or residents in Brook House.

FAR IN ADVANCE, I make the arrangements for moving day. When I arrive for the big event, I am frustrated to find that David is away on a field trip. I am reluctant to disrupt his room without his participation, but my time is limited. I decide to gamble on David's trust in me and on my having his new room comfortably organized by the time he returns. I don't want him to walk in on chaos.

Working at mach speed, I reach my goal. By the time David returns and finishes his lunch, only the picture hanging remains to be done. Holding my breath, I usher him into his new room. He is delighted.

Together we begin hanging pictures. David serves as artistic director. He is enthused about the picture montage I'm creating on one wall—a grouping patterned on the one Terry designed for his previous room. "These pictures are fabulous!" he exclaims, as if seeing them for the first time. These are the same pictures that have hung for years in his bedroom at home, and for the last four months in his room in Brook House.

"They should be fabulous, David. You're the photographer!"

"I guess you're right. I took every picture here except for the one of the men around the table. I'm in that one!" he observes.

I've just hung the last picture in the grouping. David effuses, "This is a terrific beginning. The wonderful thing is that we can add to it as we find more pictures!" Then he pauses. "No, this is probably enough; you know I'm getting pretty old, Dear."

David continues to watch and make suggestions as I hang pictures on other walls. At one point he exclaims, "Wow! You must think I'm going to be around for a while if you're going to all *this* trouble!"

Later, as I am leaving Willowglen, I pass the dining room. David is already seated with his dinner partners, Fran, Gertrude, and Elise.

Pausing to say good bye, I comment, "You all look happy as clams!"

Fran: "Exactly what does that mean, 'happy as clams'? All my life I've heard it and never known."

Me: "I've wondered about that myself, Fran. The only thing I can think of is that the two halves of a clamshell meet and form a curve that resembles an ear-to-ear grin. Can you buy that?"

Fran, nodding soberly, though without conviction: "I *think* so."

David: "I guess I've never known either, but that makes some sense."

Elise: "Well yes, uh huh. Yes, yes, uh huh, uh huh."

Gertrude: "I've never even *heard* the expression, but then I'm from Oklahoma. There's a lotta things we've never heard of in Oklahoma. In Oklahoma we say, 'happy as clowns.'"

We all agree that "happy as clowns" is more logical than "happy as clams" and that Oklahomans probably don't receive nearly enough respect.

At this point Gertrude, one of Willowglen's most functional and socially adept residents, offers, "After dinner, how 'bout I take us all out for ice cream?" Everyone at the table excitedly accepts her invitation. They begin discussing their favorite flavors and planning their orders. By the time dinner is finished, they will all have forgotten the promised ice cream. The fact that Gertrude has no car, doesn't drive, and wouldn't have a clue how to find the nearest ice cream parlor won't be an issue.

I HAVE NOTICED THAT David tends to rise (or fall) to the cerebral level of those around him. The level in Meadow House is decidedly higher than that in Brook House. Tonight there is a serenity about him that I haven't seen since before he moved to Willowglen. He seems at peace.

In the days that follow, I never observe a period of transition. Of course, I don't ask David if he is happier with this new arrangement, because he doesn't remember that he has ever lived in another area of the complex. But from everything I see, I believe David is where he belongs.

Carl

Carl is a new resident at Willowglen. He is large, probably six-foot-two and 250 pounds. Though I have never seen him behave aggressively, there is a sinister aura about Carl. His face is expressionless. His penetrating stare is unnerving. His speech is severely limited. In fact, I have heard him speak only two words.

"Hi Carl!" I greet him each time I arrive.

Long seconds pass as he holds me in his riveting gaze. Finally he responds in monotone with his two words, "Hi Carl."

Numerous times, David has warned me about Carl. "Stay away from him. He's a terrible man. I hate that guy—he scares me."

I have never heard David speak this way about another resident. I know his fear must be intense. I can see how Carl would be intimidating to him. Carl's size alone is formidable relative to David's diminutive stature.

So, David and Carl coexist—from a distance. I notice that others avoid Carl too.

AFTER ATTENDING David's quarterly evaluation, Terry is waiting for me at the door while I walk David back to his room. As we pass through the living room of Meadow House, I notice Carl, alone on a sofa. His somber eyes are fixed on us.

"Hi Carl!" I say with a big smile.

After we pass, I hear his "Hi Carl" echo.

Soon I am aware that Carl has left the sofa and is rapidly gaining on us as we approach David's room. My hand is on the doorknob when Carl reaches us. He stands so close I can feel the heat from his body on my back.

David, alarmed by Carl's overbearing presence, says in a harsh, assertive tone, "Get *away* from us! We don't *want* you here! Leave us *alone!*"

Carl hesitates momentarily before turning slowly and walking away. David and I step into his room.

"David, I can see how uncomfortable Carl makes you feel. I don't blame you for feeling the way you do. Maybe if you knew more about Carl, you wouldn't be so frightened by him. Carl has a disease that has changed his personality and destroyed his ability to speak."

In a rush of emotion, David begins to cry. "Oh no! The poor guy! How awful! I was so mean to him! I need to find him right away and tell him I'm so sorry!"

"David, I admire your compassion and your courage, but I don't think it's necessary to apologize to Carl right now. I imagine that, just like you, Carl doesn't remember things for a long time. My guess is that he has already forgotten how you treated him. Maybe next time you see Carl, you can just smile at him. That will make him feel wonderful."

Without knowing Carl's circumstances, I am hesitant to encourage David into a situation that could become combative.

I stay long enough for David to regain his composure, then hurry to meet Terry. I feel profound sadness for both David and Carl. They are locked in their separate nightmares. David will not remember to smile at Carl. Carl would not respond appropriately if David remembered. David will remain afraid. Carl will remain lonely.

Rethinking the Closet

David has been at Willowglen for five months, and he continues to express frustration with his locked closet. Now that he has settled into his new routine, I wonder if he might be able to cope with free access to his belongings. I want to give him another chance. For the second time I unlock his closet.

Two weeks pass. David deals appropriately with his regained privilege. But sometime during the third open-closet week, he reverts to his previous obsession: pulling his clothes from their hangers, blanketing his floor with them, searching for his suitcases in preparation for returning home. David has no suitcases. At the end of the third week I find the closet locked.

Gabriel García Márquez

"David, last night I was reading an old book of yours, *One Hundred Years of Solitude*, by Gabriel …"

"García Márquez," David finishes for me.

My breath catches. I wonder: *How is this possible? At times David doesn't remember that he's married, doesn't even remember Terry's name—a significant fact of his life for sixty-four years—then suddenly, Gabriel García Márquez?*

"David, of course, you know *exactly* who I'm talking about! Terry gave me a *New Yorker* article about Mr. García Márquez. The article inspired me to reread the book. Terry gave me your copy. I like reading the same book you enjoyed years ago, David."

"Yes, but if I tried to read it today, it wouldn't make one damn bit of sense to me."

"That may be true, David. Still, I am having a wonderful feeling of closeness and communion with you, as I read your book—appreciating the brilliance of your mind as it was nearly thirty years ago when you read it."

"Really? You're a great love to tell me this."

"Well, I for sure wouldn't tell you just to make you feel good. Throughout your life you have been recognized for your fine mind, David. For example, a number of your speeches are in the Western History Archives of the Denver Public Library.

"Whaaat?"

"That's right, David. The speeches you gave when you were rallying support for the Auraria Campus project are preserved at the library. And while we are addressing the subject of your brilliance, let's not forget that you were invited to be a charter member of The Literary Club."

"What Literary Club?"

"It was a long time ago, David—probably thirty years—but you were among a group of distinguished men who agreed it would be fun and mind-expanding to form a literary club. There were twelve members—one man for each month of the year. For its original

focus, the group chose English literature in the eighteenth and nine-
teenth centuries. Every month, one man would host the meeting by
providing dinner for the twelve members. The host was also responsible for choosing an appropriate topic, researching it, and presenting a scholarly paper to the membership on his appointed evening.
One topic you wrote about for The Literary Club was, 'Street Cries
of London in the Eighteenth Century.' We should go back through
your boxes of memorabilia and find 'Street Cries of London …' "

"No kidding! This is amazing. Am I still a member?"

"No, when you were eighty-five, you resigned your membership.
In your letter of resignation, you said the club had been such an
important part of your own intellectual life, you wanted to see the
club continue, and you felt its continuation depended on 'younger
and more vigorous minds.' Those were your exact words—I've read
your resignation letter, David."

"Sounds like resigning was the right thing to do."

"Yes, I think so, but it must have been a difficult decision for you
to make."

David is silent, pensive. After a long pause I continue, "But getting back to Gabriel García Márquez, David, and his book *One Hundred Years of Solitude*. It's a complex story, but you appreciated the
book from the beginning—long before García Márquez won the
Nobel Prize for it. You've always had an exceptional mind, David."

"Thank you, Dear. Now let's talk about our travel plans. How are
we going to get back to the States, and when do we leave?"

Where's My Dog Lovie?

"Where's my dog Lovie?" David asks incongruously one day.

Matter-of-factly I answer, "Lovie isn't living, David."

"Oh no! That can't be!" he protests, then immediately wants to
know how she died.

"Lovie was old, sick, and uncomfortable, so you and Terry had to
put her to sleep several years ago."

"Do they ever do that to people? Some of my friends could use it. They are really completely gone," he says, tapping his temple—his usual twinkle is absent.

Help Me Get Out of Here

"Can you help me get out of here, Dear?" David pleads. "These are not my kind of people. The people here don't read books; they don't have interesting ideas; they don't appreciate art, music, or the theater; they don't travel or even have careers. And between the two of us, I think that some of the people around here don't have all their buttons. You have to get me out of here!"

Of course, in many ways David himself precisely fits the profile he has just described. Even with his remarkable self-awareness, he doesn't realize that he is among his peers. He longs to associate with people who are more vital and dynamic. But shortly after his sad request, I witness two incidents that enable me to appreciate more fully the burden under which David labors.

Malcolm

David and I are sitting together in the living room of Meadow House when portly Malcolm, 6 feet and 225 pounds, clad only in his shorts and T-shirt—undulating within them and giggling out of them to be perfectly precise—strides boldly into the living room of Meadow House, draws up a wing-backed chair, and settles in hopefully for some social time. Proper David shoots me an "Isn't someone going to do something?" look.

An alarmed caregiver, whose accent reveals her foreign origin, rushes up to Malcolm, entreating loudly, "NO, NO, NO! Mall-coom! You no dress! You no can beeeee! COME! NOW!"

The diminutive caregiver, a five-foot featherweight, intends to single-handedly roust Malcolm from his chair. Malcolm swings a beefy arm and easily deflects his tormentor.

Undaunted, still chanting, "NO, Mallcoom! NO, Mallcoom!" she darts in for another attempt at dislodging our hero.

Sitting across the room with David, I can see that someone is about to suffer bodily harm and it's not "Mallcoom."

Quickly I step over to Malcolm's chair and speak directly but quietly into his ear: "Malcolm, you're in a public place wearing only your underwear. We like your company, but we'll enjoy your company even more if you go to your room and put some clothes on."

Genuinely surprised, Malcolm looks down at his skivvies. In one motion he lunges for a nearby afghan and wraps it around himself. Thus attired, he shuffle-trots out of the room, pursued by the caregiver who calls to me over her shoulder, "Oh tank you! Tank you!"

Effie

Another day, a resident named Effie is pitifully calling, "Sheila! Where are you, Sheila? I need you, Sheila!"

Passing through the room, the head nurse instructs Barbara, a nearby caregiver, "Sheila will be here in a few minutes. Calm Effie until Sheila arrives."

Barbara steps forward. "I'm right here!"

"*You're* not Sheila! I want *Sheila!*" Effie announces indignantly, drawing away.

"You're confused! I *am* Sheila, and I'm right here!" insists the caregiver.

Effie, now wailing, calls, "*Sheila? Sheila?* Where are you?" Effie's wailing turns to sobbing, "Shei-laaa, Shei-laaa ..."

The argument escalates into a physical as well as verbal tug-of-war as Barbara tries to maneuver the resistant Effie away from other residents while still adamantly proclaiming her false identity as Sheila.

WHAT I HAVE WITNESSED leaves me wondering how much of the belligerent, aggressive, and violent behavior attributed to those who have dementia is really a result of caregiver ineptness. No wonder David insists, "These are not my kind of people. You have to help me get out of here!"

Struggling to cope with his personal horror, David now finds himself living within a larger nightmare.

Writing a Book

"David, I'm writing a book about you."

"Whaaaat? You're kidding!"

"I'm *not* kidding, David. For a long time I have been thinking about it. So, a few days ago, I began!"

"You won't use my real name, will you?"

"Interesting you would think of that. I've thought about it too. One part of me wants very much to use your real name. You're exceptional, David. I'd like people to know this. The other part of me feels it is unthinkable to use your real name. You're entitled to your privacy."

"Yes, I agree I need my privacy."

"Then it's settled: a fictitious name."

"This book you're writing about me—I would think that the top three or four publishers in the country would want to pick it right up," he winks.

Moments later, David slips back into his fog.

ON TWO SEPARATE OCCASIONS when we discuss the book, David suggests that I not use his real name. But when I take the first draft of the manuscript to show him, he is disappointed that his name doesn't appear. Family members also encourage me to use their real names. Eventually we all agree that authentic names will be used.

When I show David a revised copy of the manuscript with his name in it, he is obviously pleased. Teasingly he asks, "Once people read the book, will I have to leave town?"

I'd Rather Kiss You

David is sitting in his room at Willowglen. The newspaper is folded in his lap. His head is bowed, and he doesn't look up when I enter.

"David?" I call softly.

Instantly alert, he cries out with emotion, "Oh my God, Darling! Where did you come from? Come over here! I'd rather kiss you than go to heaven!"

"David! What a precious and poetic thing to say to me! Is that something original you just came up with—'I'd rather kiss you than go to heaven'?"

Silently, David rises from his chair and moves to the center of his room where he stands with feet slightly apart, both hands resting on his cane planted in front of him—his typical pontificating stance. Some time has passed, and I begin to wonder: *Did he hear my question? Does he remember it now?* His brow is furrowed, and he tilts his head contemplatively to one side. The silence lengthens. Then a pleased grin beams across his face, and he replies enthusiastically, "*Yes!* I think it's original—my *own* idea!"

In all of our years together, David has never called me by my name. He doesn't even recognize my name when other people refer to me. But unfailingly, his face is a wrinkled tapestry of delight when I arrive. His original, lyrical greeting on this day has once again affirmed our bond.

A Simple Afternoon

We're out for lunch and a haircut. At some point, David uses the men's room and emerges with his fly open.

"David, just between you and me, your fly is open," I offer nonchalantly.

Quickly reaching down to zip, he grins, "I can dream, can't I?"

We're driving away from the barbershop when I comment, "David, your haircut is dynamite! You look ten years younger."

Laughing he responds, "Ten years younger is fine, but it's *still* not enough to do *us* any good!"

It's fun to see a few sparks of David's old friskiness. All afternoon there has been a flirty swagger to his demeanor. On a good day he still has plenty of spirit.

We return to Willowglen. I go through David's closet to find things that need to be mended or dry-cleaned. We visit, look at his picture album, read again the growing collection of cards he has received.

It's time for me to leave. I take David to the activity room to join a group of residents who are singing with a guest pianist. He has a hard time comprehending that I am about to leave. Finally accepting, he says, "Darling, thank you for this wonderful day. It's been a joy."

Then vague comprehension and acceptance shift to full reality, and David's expression clouds. Tears sparkle in his eyes as he haltingly chokes out the words, "I don't know whether to cry before you leave or after."

"Oh, David, I'm sad, too—always sad when I have to leave you," I say, putting my arms around him. "But our sadness at saying good-bye means there is love between us. So let's cry *whenever* we need to and hold onto the love while we're apart."

"Good idea—*very* good idea," he agrees.

I hold David for a few more moments, and without saying good-bye, I leave.

I'm a Changed Man

"Stop!" David says as we're leaving the Willowglen parking lot on our way to lunch.

"You need to know that I am a changed man, Darling—not worth a damn." Pointing to his head he says dejectedly, "I'm not all here."

"David, I understand what you're saying. Your mind is certainly not what it once was. Over the years I have witnessed your decline, Loved One. But that doesn't change my feelings for you. I see so many wonderful qualities in you, David. You are kind, generous, honest, courageous, perceptive, patient, and you know how to make me laugh! The confusion in your mind is frustrating for you, I know, but your confusion is not a problem for me. I love you just as you are, David."

Genuinely surprised, he responds, "Really? Then keep talking, Dear; I think you can help my confidence! You're bringing me right up!"

An Ordinary Nap

Waiting for David to come out of his bathroom one afternoon at Willowglen, I lie down on his bed and close my eyes. When he steps out and sees that I have made myself at home, he flings his arms wide and whoops, "Wow! This is wonderful, Dear! Lie there as long as you like—go to sleep if you want to. I'll just settle in and read my paper while you nap."

Hurriedly he takes up his newspaper and situates himself in an armchair, as if to cement the arrangement.

"Thanks, David, I could use a rest, and I can't think of a better *place* to rest than here in your cozy room with you nearby."

As David looks at his paper, I lie with my eyes closed, thinking about his thrilled reaction to finding me lying on his bed, and I realize it may be the ordinary texture of every day that holds the greatest potential for intimacy in life. Within the context of his existence at Willowglen, perhaps the casual simplicity of my napping on David's bed while he reads the newspaper feels to him like a sort of housewarming—a gesture that makes his room feel more lived in, less institutional—a confirmation that our relationship is authentic and intimate.

AGAIN I AM REMINDED that what David craves now is nothing more complicated than the warm, matter-of-fact acceptance of his current circumstances and the simple closeness of loved ones—probably not so different from what most human beings crave.

11

The Challenge of Self-Esteem

How Can I Get a Job?

"Would you be able to tell me, Dear, how can I get a job?" David asks.

"I wish I *could* tell you, David. It would make you feel terrific if you had a responsible position, wouldn't it?"

"You're darn right it would!" he agrees.

"The problem is that you're ninety-four years old, David, and you've been retired for thirty years. Business techniques have changed in those thirty years. For example, computers are now commonplace in the business world, and you have never used a computer. Another roadblock to employment is your memory. We both know that you have problems these days remembering things. A reliable memory is a necessity in today's fast-paced business environment, David."

"Yes, I guess you're right," he concedes.

"Still, you would enjoy participating and feeling that you are doing something worthwhile every day," I continue.

"That's exactly right!" he agrees.

"You're in a tough spot, David," I sympathize.

THIS IS NOT THE FIRST TIME the job issue has come up. Despite his tremendous losses, David retains his basic need for a sense of accomplishment. Over the years, we have discussed this issue. He has expressed that he misses the camaraderie—the bond that results from building a team and meeting challenges with his colleagues. He misses the satisfaction of playing a pivotal role in a successful endeavor. David has not forgotten the fulfillment of accomplishment.

The Power of Reminiscence

My years with David have given me a new appreciation for the power and importance of reminiscence. In fact, I have gained serious respect for the convention that created the stereotype of old folks sitting around, talking about the "good old days." Observing David has given me fresh insight into the role of reminiscence in our lives.

Surely others before me have figured this out, but I am convinced that as we age and become less able to go places, do things, and manifest our vitality, the more we gain our fulfillment from *remembering* our former experiences and accomplishments. However, those who experience the mental erosion of dementia are in a double bind: they can no longer do it *or* remember it. Added to David's inability to do or remember is his acute and haunting *awareness* that he cannot do or remember. Consequently, his resources for maintaining self-esteem are severely limited.

Although I am not as thoroughly versed in David's history as would be most helpful to him, I can ease him out of downward spirals by telling him stories from his life that reflect to him the glories of his prime. I serve as a human mirror that reveals the essence of his identity to him. For example, I tell him stories about the International Executive Service Corps (IESC) or his invitation to be inducted into the Colorado Business Hall of Fame. David's typical response is "Wow! Seriously? I did *that*? Ha! Not bad, huh?"

Far from being discouraged that he can't remember his own accomplishments, David is delighted to have a personal historian. He squares his shoulders and cocks his head with regained self-confidence.

THE TRAUMA OF DEMENTIA is not the simple frustration of forgetting. The trauma includes the horror of being separated from one's self, a self made up largely of one's memories. A person without access to their memories—to their essential self—can easily become overwhelmed by the terror of being alone.

As I have rebuilt my life as a single person, I have often comforted myself with the idea that even if I remain single, I will never be totally alone—I will always have myself. But unless there is someone to hold up his historical mirror for him, David doesn't have even himself. Dementia brings new meaning to the word *alone*.

International Executive Service Corps

Thirty years ago, soon after he retired, David joined the International Executive Service Corps (IESC), a group of outstanding businesspeople from around the world. Participants in IESC donate their time as consultants and live for extended periods in assigned countries. They work side by side with their hosts, teaching them effective business techniques. In his capacity as an IESC member, David, always accompanied by Terry, had nine assignments, was involved in numerous successful projects, and made lasting friendships around the world.

Many of the pictures on David's walls were taken during this period of extensive travel to faraway places. He recalls none of it. He stubbornly objects to the idea that he has been retired for thirty years, accepting this fact only after he himself does the math. Only occasionally does David sense the passage of time: For example, he will slip into a frenzy, fearing that he has been fired for having missed so much work. But David enjoys hearing about his participation in the IESC—being reminded that he traveled to interesting places and made a difference in people's lives.

Colorado Business Hall of Fame

We are on our way to the airport to meet David's daughter, Sissy, who is coming from New York for a weekend visit. As we drive along, I give David another reflection from his past.

"Years ago, David, you were named as an inductee to the Colorado Business Hall of Fame. The purpose of the Hall of Fame is to honor business leaders who have made significant contributions to private enterprise and who have served as business role models to young people. Never a glory seeker, you declined the honor. Gene Amole, a columnist for the *Rocky Mountain News*, documented this story about you in a column headlined 'Humble Hero Served Us Well.'"

Still driving, I tell David the essence of the following excerpt from Mr. Amole's newspaper column.

> When man bites dog, that's news. It is also news when David Touff won't be inducted into the Colorado Business Hall of Fame … because he says he doesn't deserve the honor. In today's award-happy society, humility is a rare virtue …
>
> For Touff, retailing was high drama. He believed in the quality of his merchandise. He treated customers and employees with respect. He saw the department store as a focal point for American living, and he wanted to make it as appealing and as helpful as possible.
>
> David Touff was the best at what he did. I am sorry that modesty prevents him from accepting the recognition he so richly deserves. Young merchants would do well to emulate the qualities that led to his success.
>
> Dave, I just want you to know there are a lot of us out here who appreciated your commitment to service and to the quality of the products you sold. You have always been one of my heroes.*

"So, David, they wanted to honor you, but you turned it down."

"Wow! No kidding? I wouldn't turn it down today," he chuckles. "If they gave me another shot, I'd take it! I could really use it now, Dear. Now that I'm … what's the word … oh I can't … what am I trying to … you see, that's the problem … not up … what's the … not up?"

"Down?" I offer.

"Yes, down, but even more."

"Discouraged, David?"

"That's it, discouraged. What were we talking about, Dear?"

---

*"Humble hero served us well," by Gene Amole, *Rocky Mountain News*, Jan. 16, 1990, p. 7. Reprinted with permission of the *Rocky Mountain News*.

"The Colorado Business Hall of Fame—the award that you turned down years ago."

"Yes! Well, it would boost me up now."

The Purpose of Life

A year and a half before he moved to Willowglen, I asked, "What is the purpose of life, David?"

Not hesitating, he answered, "The purpose of life, of *my* life anyway, is contribution. It is important for me to give something, to believe that I add something, to know that in some way I make a difference."

More than two years have passed when I ask again, "David, what is the purpose of life?"

Pensively, slowly, he answers, "Joy ... learning ... and the affection of others."

"I like that, David!"

Then I relate our earlier conversation on the subject, and David replies animatedly, "Oh that's *good*! Contribution! Yes, I'll go with that!"

12

Acceptance and Relationships

I Live Here Now

Since the day David moved to Willowglen, there has been a dominant two-part theme to all of our conversations. We may digress briefly to Gabriel García Márquez, the pictures on the wall, places he has been, people he has known. But reliably, we always return to "Where's Terry, and when are we going home?"

David has been at Willowglen for nine months. One day when I visit him he says earnestly, "This place is not at all like home, but they do a pretty good job here. Don't try to get in, though. I don't think you'd like it."

When I see him again two days later, he states offhandedly, "You know I live here now."

After nine months, a breakthrough! David has acknowledged that he won't be returning home. Of course he'll need to be reminded. Still, I interpret his acknowledgment as the beginning of acceptance.

Postcards and Old Friends

At least twice a week I visit David at Willowglen. Each encounter with him further affirms the respect I have for my courageous friend. Between visits, I make it a point to call him. On the phone, he is never quite sure who I am, but a phone call is another reminder that someone loves him and is thinking of him.

Still convalescing and emotionally depleted, Terry visits infrequently, but she has begun a postcard campaign. Several times a week, she writes to David. He has amassed a sizeable collection that he reads repeatedly. These cards are a ubiquitous fixture in the pockets of his sport coats, in scrambled corners of dresser drawers, Kleenex boxes, Dopp kit, medicine cabinet, and every possible but unlikely cranny. Terry's correspondence effort is making a significant difference in David's sense of ease and calm.

David's son visits him every weekend, and his daughter in New York writes faithfully. David's amazingly steadfast friends come to see him often.

Recently, a longtime friend and business associate of David's turned ninety-nine. Knowing that David wouldn't be able to attend the party, his friends brought the party to him at Willowglen: seven aging men, led by the tottering, ninety-nine-year-old birthday boy himself, arrived with cake, candles, and high spirits.

Friendship like this is not common. It is cultivated over years of respect. This remarkable gesture by his friends is testimony to David's character and the exemplary life he has lived.

But Do They Love Me?

David's attitude has been upbeat, but in a two-week period I have noticed a dramatic decline in his communication skills and attention span. He seems flighty and unable to participate in my simplest attempts at conversation with him.

I feel that David has reached a stage where his awareness is diminished, but blessedly his emotional pain has lessened too. His frenzied chatter leads nowhere. I get the feeling that he is trying to be my host, to entertain me. But he lacks all context and the ability to follow a single thought to its conclusion. Maybe this chatter is another form of masking. Maybe it's panicking—a monumental effort to stay connected as he feels his mental grip loosening. But whatever the origin of this new behavior, David is consistently in good humor. David's previous feelings of anxiousness and discouragement with himself, for now at least, are absent.

David has been at Willowglen for almost a year. I long for our times together to be comforting and fulfilling for him, but I have no way of gauging if they are. His speech and behavior are so disjointed and scattered I can't be sure my presence brings him any joy, but I'm thankful he doesn't seem particularly distressed.

Toward the end of our visit, David points to the framed "Reminders" on his dresser. For the first time all day he speaks coherently.

"I want you to take a look at that, Dear. It's terrific!"

"I'm glad you like it, David. I wrote it for you."

"No kidding? Why did you do that?"

"I thought it might help you when you feel confused."

"Well it sure does help me—about ten times every day! Read it to me, will you, Darling?"

I start down the list. Near the end I read, "David's wife, Terry, and his two children, Michael and Sissy, care deeply for David."

David interrupts, "Yes, but do they *love* me?"

"They certainly do, David!" I quickly reassure him.

"Then it should *say* they love me, and that should be right at the *top* of the page!"

Unbelievable! This, in such sharp contrast to what I have witnessed for the past hour. I am stunned. "David, you need a revised copy of this sheet. I'll bring it when I come to see you on Tuesday."

THE OBLIVION THAT PERVADES David's world has not lessened his need for love or his need to have his relationship to his loved ones accurately defined. I see it as a measure of his enduring self-esteem that he insists his relationship to his family be headlined and stated in the most positive terms.

13

One Step Forward, Two Steps Back

Beckos on My Elbows

David has been at Willowglen for over a year. His verbal expression has reached a new low, and his comprehension seems severely limited. At times dialogue with David is hardly possible, because he can't remember from the beginning to the end of a sentence what we are talking about.

"Weren't we ... well ... wasn't it ... wasn't it ... a woman maybe ... no ... Ireland, that's it, Ireland ... a gift, yes, in my jar ... the traveling Mexican magic show ... for pictures ... sometime ... not dark ... oh, hell."

"David, let's start again. I want to understand what you're trying to tell me."

"Well, there was the guy ... twelve beckos ... beckos ... too far."

"Beckos?"

"Yes, beckos, on my elbows." David holds up both hands to show me deep, angry-looking cracks at the corners of his thumbs.

"Oh, David, these look terribly painful. Let's put some lotion on them immediately. I'm also going to give you a big glass of water to drink. Believe it or not, water will help."

Not long after this, in a Japanese restaurant, our food has just been served. I add soy sauce to David's bowl of rice and mix it in.

Before I have a chance to put soy sauce on my own rice, David comments, "My cheese suit is better than yours."

"What's that, David? I don't understand."

"My cheese suit!" he says, scowling and jabbing his finger toward his rice.

"Oh, your rice is a different color from mine?"

"Yes!" he says, frustrated.

"Your rice is brown, because I put soy sauce on it for you. My rice is white, because I haven't added soy sauce to my rice yet."

"Why didn't you say so?" he demands.

I IMAGINE A high-speed ticker tape of knowledge coursing through David's mind; he randomly seizes any word or fragment of an idea that flickers by, regardless of its relevance to what he is trying to say.

Does David assume that anything he seizes from the ticker is relevant? Does he believe he has expressed what is on his mind? Is anything on his mind? Is he surprised when others don't comprehend—when they dismiss him as deficient, or subject him to the challenge of translating? Does he feign indignation to cover his lack of understanding? Does he still have understanding? Is he simply unable to find the right words to express his thoughts? Do random words just spill out, motivated by nothing more than the habit of talking? These unanswerable questions haunt me.

I spend a lot of time saying, "Take your time, David. We'll figure it out. I remember where we started. We'll go back to the beginning if we need to."

Regrouping

One day at Willowglen, Anna, an extraordinary caregiver, discreetly tells me that David is becoming a problem. He is staying up until the early morning hours, restlessly pacing the halls. On two occasions when caregivers have tried to coax him to put on his nightshirt and go to bed, he has struck them with his cane. When David tires of pacing—two or three hours before breakfast—he insists on sleeping in his clothes.

If this problem is not addressed, I fear he will soon be viewed as unmanageable. He may even be asked to leave Willowglen. The next stop after Willowglen would be far more institutional: linoleum floors, fluorescent lights, two residents to a hospital-style room, more regimentation, and behavior-modifying drugs if necessary.

I believe that a lack of daytime stimulation is disrupting David's sleep pattern. He dozes during the day. At night he is alert, not ready for sleep. When pressured by caregivers to go to bed at a conventional hour, he becomes aggressive. Further, I suspect that his daytime exhaustion is giving the appearance of dramatic mental decline. It is also obvious to me that he is suffering from significant dehydration. I am convinced that dehydration is a major contributing factor to David's sudden, *apparent* deterioration.

While all of these possibilities may be impacting on David's situation, it may also be that he is in natural, irrevocable decline. Whatever the cause of his difficulties, I want to help him if I can.

Willowglen offers a wide range of activities, including many field trips. David has never been an enthusiastic participant. I believe that he is not being stimulated in ways that meet his needs. By his own admission, David is depressed by the other residents. He craves interaction with people who are more functional.

Although I have taken David to his various appointments, it has been my habit to visit with him at Willowglen rather than venture out with him on excursions. In his early days at Willowglen, before he was well adjusted to his new environment, outings were unsettling for him. Reflecting, I realize that our recent outings have actually been enjoyable. Maybe David needs to spend more time in the outside world.

On the Road Again

After Anna speaks to me about David, I go to his room and find him sitting in a chair, asleep. He is only mildly pleased to see me, and too groggy to look at the book I have brought to show him. He appears extremely dehydrated. I quickly cancel my other appointments for the afternoon with the intention of devoting as much time to David as he needs.

I suggest that we go for a ride. He is not interested. While he nods in and out of consciousness, I ply him with water, comb his hair, and give him a shave. Gradually, he rallies.

"David, let's drive to the Cherry Creek Mall. You need new hand-kerchiefs—maybe a few other things too. After we shop, we can have dinner together in a restaurant. What do you think?"

"I think, when do we leave?" David says, pushing out of his chair.

On our way out of Willowglen, I quickly key in the five-digit exit code on the touch pad. David exclaims, "Wow! You have impressive hands—very nimble fingers!"

Nimble fingers? Already we're making progress. Twenty minutes ago, David was in a stupor!

Driving toward town, I talk to David about his situation.

"David, I've heard that you're having trouble sleeping at night. You're spending a lot of nighttime hours walking the halls. In the daytime, you can't stay awake to participate in activities."

With good-humored, mock bravado, he responds, "Yeah right, I'm just too high up to spend my days with everyone else."

David means to be amusing, but he has touched on a truth. From his perspective, he is among an intelligent minority within a mentally deficient population. As I have observed in the past, he is able to discern the deficiencies of others, but not always his own. How human of him!

As we drive along, David begins to speak, he hesitates, then mumbles unintelligibly. I reach over and put my hand on his knee, "David, I believe you know what you want to say, but you seem to be having trouble finding the words to express your thoughts."

This small encouragement helps him regain his equilibrium, and he responds, "That's *exactly* right! God, I'm glad you know me so well."

At the mall David is reborn. Although confused and sometimes socially inappropriate in his offhanded interactions with strangers, he is curious, surprisingly perceptive, and quite articulate. Ever the merchant, David is interested in the display, the volume, and the quality of the merchandise. He comments on the diversity and number of shoppers. He even wants to know what time it is and what day of the week so he can determine if there are enough shoppers for the time slot. "If it's 10:30 Tuesday morning, there are enough people here. If it's 2 o'clock Saturday afternoon, this place is in trouble!"

Our shopping complete, we stroll, still indoors, into the common area of the mall. We sit near a large play arena designed for toddlers. Amused by the children, David comments enthusiastically on their limber acrobatics and adorable interactions with each other.

The theme of this arena is an oversized breakfast. The play structures resemble eight-foot-diameter cereal bowls filled with king-sized pillows of shredded wheat garnished with strawberries and blueberries the size of melons, French toast and bacon strips too large for Paul Bunyan, and fried eggs as big as semi-truck tires. As we sit observing, I wonder if David grasps the theme.

"David, have you noticed that all of the play structures are gigantic replicas of breakfast food?"

He stares at me blankly.

"See the French toast and the enormous bowls of cereal—and over there, the ten-foot banana?"

"Whaaaat?" he responds irritably.

Wishing I had been content with simple toddler-watching, I continue with little hope of David's grasping what I want him to see. "See that big thing right there that looks like a giant piece of bacon?"

For no apparent reason, the puzzle shifts into place. David yelps gleefully, "Well for God's sake! Fan*tastic*! This is the best thing I've ever seen! Whoever came up with this idea was a genius!"

Now he watches the shenanigans with even greater interest.

DURING OUR YEARS of adventuring, I've observed that David finds his greatest clarity, comfort, and fulfillment not in his rare, poignant insights, but in the simplicity of the present moment. He appreciates the warmth of the sunshine, the taste and texture of the food, the beautiful dress worn by the woman at the next table, an animated child, a dog loping across the park without its leash.

Many of the things David noticed in the past, he no longer notices. How perfect that being with him has heightened my sense of awareness, so now, as he declines, I am able to guide his focus and stimulate his interest in those things he is still able to appreciate.

AFTER HALF AN HOUR of the preschool floorshow, we're ready to look for a restaurant. David suggests "a place that will have a good hamburger and fries, apple pie, and a cup of coffee!"

We quickly find the qualifying eatery.

Sitting in the reception area waiting for our table, I comment, "Isn't this bench we're sitting on unusually high, David?"

He shoots back with a grin, "Yes, and just think how it feels to a little guy like me! My feet are dangling in thin air—a foot above the ground!"

When our food arrives, David moans, "Too much food! This will be embarrassing! I'll never be able to eat all this!" Then he voraciously consumes every morsel.

It is dark when we return to Willowglen. David is in good spirits after a full afternoon and evening. I continue to wear him out until 7:45: trimming his fingernails, straightening the pictures on his bedroom walls, and sorting out the clothes in his closet that need to be dry-cleaned.

Next morning, I call Anna. The strategy has worked. David has slept through the night (in his nightshirt) for the first time in several weeks.

Looks like we're back to square one, or maybe it's square two. Years ago, we were wide-eyed adventure seekers. Now we are seasoned travelers.

Water

From the beginning of our association, I have observed that the simple intake of water improves David's demeanor and mental clarity. Among certain health-conscious individuals, water has long been touted as a cure-all. Observing David's physical responses to water, I have become convinced that the water advocates are on to something.

It is fact that water is the single most abundant substance in the human body, accounts for about two-thirds of an adult's body weight, and virtually all chemical reactions occurring in the body depend upon water. It is also widely known that as human beings age, they tend toward dehydration, and dehydration manifests negatively in every system of the body—from decreased digestive function to sluggish cerebral function.

Water is so vital to human function that human beings can survive far longer without food than without water. Yet this elemental, affordable substance, crucial for optimal health, is widely overlooked in the care of the elderly.

Although water disguised as punch, tea, coffee, soda, etc., is better than no fluid at all, these drinks put an added stress on the body to filter out the disguises before the water can do its job. And ironically, beverages containing sugar actually leach water from the body's cells, thereby increasing dehydration.

In short, there is no substitute for water—pure and simple.

David's Signs of Dehydration

In conjunction with David's recent decline, I have observed his significant dehydration. Without fail, when I arrive to take David out, his lips are chapped and sticking to his teeth, his mouth sounds sticky when he speaks, his face is drawn, his eyes are dull, his skin is dry, and his color is ashen. Deep, angry fissures have developed at the corners of David's thumbs and several of his fingers. These cracks heal within a number of days of maintained hydration. Of course, appropriate water intake must continue or the cracks will reappear.

I now carry bottled water in the car for David. Before we even drive away from Willowglen, he is drinking water. Invariably he comments, "My God, that's a good drink! What is that?"

David doesn't ask for water. I offer it. I always tell him that his drinking water will help him to think more clearly. Given this information, he drinks enthusiastically. Within five minutes of his initial water intake, David's appearance, attitude, and mental clarity improve. In the course of a four-hour outing, David will drink at least a quart of water.

Confirming my observation that adequate hydration is critical for David, I recently saw a relevant, four-column, public-service announcement in one of Denver's major dailies. Sponsored by the Colorado Department of Health Care Policy and Financing, Colorado Department of Public Health and Environment, and the American Association of Retired Persons, the announcement was headlined "Proper Hydration Is Essential in Older Adults." The announcement included the following list of warning signs:

- Drinking less than six cups of liquid per day
- Having trouble swallowing liquids
- Needing help when drinking from a cup or glass
- Confusion/fatigue
- The presence of dry mouth, cracked lips, and sunken eyes

WITH TERRY'S BLESSING, I begin to take David out at least four days a week. I have a four-point agenda: (1) Change David's sleep pattern with daytime stimulation. (2) Give David frequent respite from his Willowglen peers. (3) Provide David with more opportunities to interact with fully functioning people. (4) Rehydrate David.

Subsequent field trips are as successful as the first, though not always without emotional tugs. After one five-hour outing, we return in time for David to eat dinner at Willowglen. Before leaving him, I help him into his chair at the dinner table. He mumbles something I can't hear. When I question him he says, "I've decided I don't need to say that."

I press him to repeat himself.

Finally, David looks up at me with tears in his eyes. "I said, 'I don't know how I can live the life that's ahead of me.'"

OCCASIONAL MOMENTS OF despair notwithstanding, David is definitely making a comeback. Our excursions are more modest than they once were. Usually they include lunch or dinner, perhaps a drive downtown, and the exploration of one store. A favorite store is Cost Plus. Seeing the exotic imports triggers David's vague memories of world travel.

With renewed stimulation, David is consistently experiencing his trademark flashes of brilliance. And from a social standpoint, traveling with him is easier than it was before he moved to Willowglen. He seems less inclined than he once was to make loud, inappropriate, public pronouncements. Perhaps now he doesn't notice the things that used to inspire his comments. When I sense that he is veering in an awkward direction, I don't hesitate to say discreetly, "This is not an appropriate conversation for us to have in public, David," or "We need to keep our voices down, because we're making a spectacle of ourselves" or "Pointing at people makes them feel uncomfortable, David." I am never accusatory, just matter-of-fact. When I guide him in this way he seems surprised, but is usually compliant.

There are exceptions. We are leaving a restaurant when David plants himself in the doorway.

"Hey, wait a minute! I want to get a card so I can bring Terry back here."

"You have a card, David. It's in your billfold. I saw you put it there not five minutes ago," I offer, hoping to end the delay.

"No, I don't remember getting a card. Let me check," he says, patting himself down, looking for his billfold.

By now there are other patrons waiting to enter the restaurant and two behind us waiting to exit.

"David," I whisper. "We need to move along. We're blocking the entrance and all eyes are on us."

"Let 'em look!" he invites loudly. "Maybe they'll decide to make a movie, and we'll all be famous!"

Nearby witnesses seem amused and accepting of an old man's eccentricity.

A Valentine

We are eating lunch in a restaurant when David overhears someone say, "Valentine's Day."

Instantly he says, "Valentine's Day—isn't that February fourteenth?"

"That's right, David!" I reply, amazed.

"What is today?"

"Today is February twelfth."

"My God, I don't think I have anything for Terry. Can you help me find something for Terry—something really great?" he pleads anxiously.

"Good idea, David! We'll go shopping as soon as we finish lunch."

David chooses a densely flowered cyclamen plant in the Day-Glo magenta color that always attracts him, then he spies a red, Mylar, helium-filled heart that he can't resist. Finally, he insists on buying chocolates.

"Chocolate is a must! Not just any chocolate—something really good," he insists.

So we go to Godiva, and he chooses exactly what he wants—no help from me, thank you very much!

And he buys a card that says, "I am incredibly particular. And you are particularly incredible!" David reads the card so many times, I am sure it will look like a hand-me-down by the time Terry receives it. Shakily, he writes "Terry" on the card and envelope. He employs my steadier hand to write his dictated sentiment inside the card. "To the best wife a guy ever had. I love you always." Then he signs his own nearly illegible name.

I promise to deliver his gifts to Terry on Valentine's Day. Not only is David thoroughly satisfied with his purchases, he is obviously uplifted by his feeling of accomplishment—a feeling that he has not experienced in months.

ON VALENTINE'S DAY, I visit David and take him a few festive tokens. One trinket I give him is a button for his lapel.

"Hey, wait a minute! What does this say?"

I read it aloud: "I am loved."

"Well, I'll have to think about this. Maybe I don't want to give certain people the idea that I'm out of the running," he teases.

You're a *Schmeichler*

"Hi, my name is Brad," our waiter says as he escorts us to our table. "I'll be taking care of you today."

"Hi, Brad, my name is Marilyn. This is my good friend, David."

"May I bring you two something to drink for starters?"

"Thanks, Brad. David needs a pot of hot water, half a cup of decaf, and a straw. I'd like a large glass of unsweetened grapefruit juice."

As Brad hurries away, David says, "Wow! Are you ever the schmeichler!"

"What's a schmeichler, David?"

"I thought you'd probably ask me, but I wish you hadn't. I'm not sure it's a word!" he says, laughing.

"Well, even if it's not a *real* word, what did you *mean* when you called me a schmeichler?"

"Oh ... someone who smiles a lot ... gets what she wants by being charming!"

"Hmmm ... sounds to me like a schmeichler may be scheming and manipulative, David. Is a used car salesman a schmeichler?"

"Well ... maybe ... yes ... a little ... but I don't think I know what I'm talking about. We never spoke a word of Yiddish in my family when I was growing up. I heard my grandmother speak it a little, but only at her house."

"That doesn't surprise me, David. Your mother and father were still children when their families came to the United States to escape the Russian pogroms. When you were a child, your family was the only Jewish family in a small rural community."

"That was Freeland, Michigan," he volunteers.

"Yes, Freeland, that's right. Well, given your parents' own harsh, early history, maybe they wanted to keep a low Jewish profile. Not speaking Yiddish was one way to keep a low profile."

Leaning toward me across the table, David says in a hushed, almost conspiratorial voice, "My God, how did you know that? That's exactly how it was!"

"It was a guess, David. I know a little about your family history. I imagined the rest."

"It's wonderful you know these things about me, Dear."

Not long after this conversation with David, I ask a Jewish friend of mine who teaches college-level Hebrew if he knows of a Yiddish word, schmeichler. He says it is not a Yiddish word, but the German word, schmeichl, means "to smile and to charm." Adding "er" could create David's word, schmeichler—one who schmeichls—one who smiles and charms.

OVER THE YEARS OF my association with David, many people have asked me, "Don't you get bored?" or "Considering all the hours you spend with David, what can you possibly find to talk about?"

Boredom has never been a problem. Finding things to talk about is no more complicated than simply responding to David, staying abreast of his own curiosity, or noticing and wondering aloud about the mysteries around us. And I often wonder if challenging David's intellect with rich conversation has slowed his decline or only made it more bearable.

OUT OF CONTEXT, the snippets of David's charm and fleeting insight can be misleading. On a good day, in the span of a three-hour outing, David may experience a total of only thirty coherent minutes. The remainder of the time I spend trying to distill meaning from David's disconnected words or easing him out of his mental tangle.

Although our frequent outings have boosted David's morale and normalized his sleeping patterns, I know that his improvement can't be sustained indefinitely. Without question, David is declining. At age ninety-four, it is only realistic to believe that his decline will accelerate.

Another May

In May 2000, I accompany Terry on a two-week trip to compensate for the trip she missed in the spring of 1999. We both feel painfully conflicted: concerned that David will be sad and confused by our absence, and guilty for abandoning him. Yet I feel supportive of Terry's need for pleasure and fulfillment in the years that are left to her.

Terry fears not only that David will feel confused and sad she is traveling so far away from him, but angry that he's being excluded from our trip. She chooses not to discuss our plans with him. However, we agree that the uniqueness of my relationship with David allows me to take a different approach from Terry's. So I write a letter to David with the understanding that I won't mention Terry's name—her only desire being to spare him hurt.

Knowing that David looks at his picture album many times each day, I leave my letter there for him, hopeful that he will read it repeatedly while we are away. Of course, I have no way of knowing if he will even sense my absence, but I feel it's appropriate to at least offer him an explanation he can ignore if it is meaningless. I attach pictures of the two of us together, so he will remember who I am. The letter helps me—it may or may not help David. At the very least, I believe he can feel the love my letter expresses.

(*I include the letter here only to demonstrate my belief that one who has dementia may, at any given moment, have the capability to receive and understand complex information.*)

May 29, 2000

Dear David,

This letter is to remind you that I am on a trip. Usually, I come to see you at least four times a week, David. While I'm away, I thought you might wonder why I am not coming to visit with you and take you to lunch.

I am leaving on May 29, 2000. I will return to Denver, late on the night of June 14. I will see you as soon as I can after my return, David—probably on June 16. To remind you of our friendship, I am also including pictures of the two of us together. While I am away, please, don't think I have forgotten you. That could *never* happen, David! You are permanently in my heart, and often in my thoughts.

While I am traveling, your dear friend and former secretary, Liz Waggener, will be visiting you regularly. I fear that after two weeks in Liz's good company, returning to my ordinary companionship will seem pretty ho-hum! Try not to forget me in favor of another woman! ☺

Below is my travel itinerary:

May 29	Fly from Denver to New York.
May 30–31	Fly from New York to Barcelona, Spain (Princesa Sofia Hotel).
May 31–June 3	Explore Barcelona, Spain.
June 3	Sail from Barcelona, Spain.
June 4	At sea.
June 5	Malaga, Spain.
June 6	Gibraltar, United Kingdom.
June 7	Cadiz, Spain.
June 8	Lisbon, Portugal (Four Seasons Hotel, Ritz).
June 8–11	Explore Lisbon, Portugal.
June 11	Fly from Lisbon to New York.
June 11–14	Visit my daughter in New York.
June 14	Fly to Denver.
June 15	Unpack, develop pictures from trip, recover from jet lag, readjust to Denver altitude.
June 16	Visit David!!!

David, my photography skills are not in the same league with yours, but I will do my amateur's best to take some pictures that we can look at together when I return.

If the international postal system works well, you will be receiving many communiqués from me while I am away. If the mail is sluggish, you will receive my postcards *after* I return. Either way, I'll drop my cards to you into the fastest mailboxes!

Please remember, David, that you are loved by many people. Terry, Michael, Sissy, and I love you immensely. There are others, too numerous to mention, who also love you and respect the exemplary life you have lived. David, when you and I are together, I often remind you of the love that constantly flows in your direction. In my absence, I have left this letter. I hope when you read this letter you will be reminded of how much you are loved.

Until I see you on June 16, David, I will carry you in my heart across the ocean.

Plenty of love,
Marilyn

DAVID FARES BEAUTIFULLY in our absence, and isn't unusually over-joyed by my return. It is good for me to learn that I am dispensable.

14

One Year, Many Losses

Realities

Now, well into his ninety-fifth year, David is still relatively strong physically, but he has lost significant ground. Constant disorientation, almost complete loss of verbal skills, and more frequent and severe TIAs are the most glaring hallmarks of his recent decline. David's high level of anxiety when we leave Willowglen makes outings counterproductive. We have given up our adventures.

The Importance of "Reminders"

We are approaching the second anniversary of David's move to Willowglen. At Terry's house one evening, David's son, Michael, and I are having a casual conversation when he volunteers, "One of the best things you've ever done for Father is that 'Reminders' list. When you sent me the list, I had some reservations. It felt almost harsh—so straightforward about dementia and how Father would be living permanently at Willowglen. But I decided to go along with it, and it's turned out to be a great thing."

"Michael, thanks. I'm thrilled if you feel the list is helpful! But I'm interested to know what changed your feelings about it—how did you move from hesitant to enthusiastic?"

Michael has a ready response. "Almost every time I visit Father, he shows me the 'Reminders.' He seems glad to have the information, but the list is more than just information for him. Most of the time he wants to read the list out loud to me. Even though he's lost most of his capacity for original speech, he can still read words. He seems pleased with himself for being able to verbalize by reading those important words to me—like he's coherently telling me something significant about himself. Evidently he understands those short sentences. I like how each simple sentence is a complete statement about his situation, but the sentences build on each other to paint a whole picture. Once he's read the list, we have a starting place for our 'conversation,' because I can go back to the reminders and enlarge on any one statement. So it helps me too."

My own experience with the reminders is similar to Michael's. Repeatedly, David produces the list and reads it to me. Sometimes we focus on it for most of an entire visit. And anytime David is confused or disbelieving when I answer his questions about where he lives and why, I turn to the list. Reading it together has never failed to calm his anxiety. As it did on the day he moved to Willowglen, the list seems to serve as an objective validation of what I am saying. Being able to see in writing the concise, matter-of-fact explanation of his situation diffuses David's anger toward me for being the bearer of bad news. But the importance of the list is difficult to quantify. Somehow it empowers David, gives him authority, lets *him* be the one to tell *us* he has a problem, rather than the other way around. David has expanded the value of the reminders well beyond what I originally anticipated.

In Maudie's Bed

Just before dinnertime one evening, I arrive at Willowglen. David is not in his room. Systematically I begin looking in the nooks where I often find him. He seems to have vanished. I enlist the help of a staff member, and we begin checking the rooms of other residents.

Dinner is well under way, we've opened many doors, and still David eludes us. I try to calm myself, but my anxiety is rising. Behind one of the few remaining doors, we find David asleep in Maudie's hand-carved, antique bed—sans Maudie. Slack-jawed, he rasps rhythmically, contentedly, under her down comforter. David hasn't lost his penchant for the aesthetically pleasing. He has inarguably chosen the most elegant bed at Willowglen for a late-afternoon siesta. His neatly folded clothes lie on a nearby chair; his socks are tucked into his perfectly parallel shoes under the bed.

Thankful that Maudie is at dinner and oblivious to her intruder, I urgently coax David toward consciousness and hurriedly help him dress. Initially he is resistant, but as we scramble I persist in explaining that he has been sleeping in Maudie's bed. Eventually he gets it and responds with hearty guffaws interspersed with nonsensical sputterings. As we laugh together, David affects the stealthy demeanor of a cat burglar. Taking his cue, I join him and we hunch furtively out of unsuspecting Maudie's room.

Although David's verbal skills often fail him, his sense of humor and his ability to laugh at himself remain. My heart sends a silent message: *David, I know you're in there.*

Saving Graces: Touch and Music

Losing the ability to converse might not have the same impact on a man less gregarious than David. But the slow, discouraged shake of his head, the flinging, dismissive wave of his hand that sketches futility in the air, the resigned slope of his shoulders—all of these indicators scream silently to me that he feels his loss deeply.

Always the genial host, David seems to believe that my visits require him to entertain me with inspired conversation. Though utterly incapable of sustained dialogue, he relentlessly aggravates and embarrasses himself by attempting it.

Sensing David's yearning for connectedness, I call upon my skills as a massage therapist. I question how effective full body massage would be for one as impaired as David—too disorienting, too invasive—but we have settled into a routine that suits our purpose. Fully clothed, David sits in an armchair. I put two bed pillows on his lap to support and cushion his arms. Stepping behind his chair, I massage his head, neck, shoulders, and upper arms. He leans his head back against my body and I massage his face. Eventually, I kneel on the floor in front of his chair, massaging lotion into his hands and forearms. When time permits, I massage his feet and lower legs. Transported, David exudes serenity. In these moments he transcends his need to speak. Even without words he has connected with another human being—one who aches to know his realities.

Still, I long to facilitate David's need to speak, less for the sake of communication than for his self-esteem. Music proves to be an instrument of fulfillment. Pirating a couple of songbooks from the activity room, we warble as we once did, this time behind the closed doors of David's room: "Tea for Two," "Girl of My Dreams," "The Sidewalks of New York," and on and on. Cued by the songbook, it all comes back. David is carried along by the familiarity of the words and melodies he mastered decades ago. But singing serves a greater purpose than whiling away an afternoon. Framed in a small window of time, David experiences the joy of forming words and combining them into meaning. Judging by the spirited way he delivers each line, he sees himself as an accomplished and articulate human being once again. Singing literally puts words into David's mouth.

Questioning "Loss of Dignity"

David's daughter, Sissy, is in town for the weekend. Though we have been communicating and she knew what to expect, she is deeply saddened to see firsthand the realities of David's condition. His deficits are orders of magnitude worse than when she saw him only two months ago. Our visiting eventually leads to contemplating loss of dignity at the end of life. I am surprised by my initial lack of feeling on the subject. Sissy returns to New York, but the questions we've raised stay with me.

At first I feel somewhat guilty for my lack of emotion regarding the loss of dignity. In the process of trying to reconcile this absence of feeling, I realize that *never*, through TIAs, bouts of diarrhea, social awkwardness, occasional rages, fading intellect, or loss of language, have I ever had the sense that David has *lost* his dignity. So I have no feelings of grief for David in this regard. My only feelings of sadness for David are similar to those I had on a recent night when I saw a tattered, lame-footed old fox make his way unsteadily across an urban street and into the underbrush that borders the interstate: overwhelming primal rushes of tenderness and melancholy, a deep longing to intervene, and a certainty that I could not. But even these feelings are simultaneously balanced by my deep respect for a living being who, imbued with the miraculous life force, moves resolutely toward his destiny. Loss of dignity? No.

Dignity, to me, means honoring and esteeming my self. Contemplating the idea of dignity, I realize I have always believed that dignity comes from within. I have never imagined that dignity is bestowed from without or dependent on the judgment of others. If, in the face of whatever life hands me, I can retain a belief in my essential worthiness, I have not lost my dignity.

But "loss of dignity" has become a hackneyed phrase in the end-of-life lexicon—perhaps, for many people, a catchall for the apprehensions they harbor regarding their own eventual decline. I wonder what the expression "loss of dignity" really means. If I trip and fall down on the sidewalk, have I lost my dignity? Maybe I've lost it only if I *think* I have. If I lie on the ground laughing at how funny I must have looked as I flailed to the ground, maybe I *haven't* lost it. If I lie on the sidewalk, beating my fists on the concrete, raging at the idiot who failed to repair the uneven slab I tripped on, have I lost my dignity? Onlookers might say I have lost it, but how would they know? It's *my* dignity. If venting my emotion is an effective catharsis and I am content with my behavior, maybe my dignity is intact. Does simply being embarrassed cause a loss of dignity? Does showing various signs of humanness such as crying or yahooing exuberantly cause one to lose dignity? If beauty is in the eye of the beholder, maybe dignity is in the eye or mind or heart of the holder—the possessor of dignity.

In Bill Moyers's TV series, *On Our Own Terms*, one man in the early stages of Lou Gehrig's disease contemplates his eventual death.

He discusses the point at which he might find his situation so intolerable he would take measures to end his life. He is adamant in his declaration that when he can no longer clean himself after defecating, he will have lost so much dignity that life will not be worth living. When that day comes, he is disappointed and frustrated, but he readily adjusts to his new level of dependency. Next, he asserts that when he can no longer feed himself, the level of indignity will be unbearable and he will definitely be ready to end his life. When his wife eventually has to feed him, he again experiences the challenge of adjustment, but he sees that life is still worth living. When all of his worst fears are realized, he finds that he has not only the genuine longing but also the inner strength to continue living. This man's essential dignity is defined *not* by his ability or inability to clean or feed himself, but by his life-affirming desire to persevere and his inner strength to do so.

A baby, in its unawareness, is not considered undignified when his diaper is being changed or when he is being fed. Have I lost my dignity if, in a state of dementia-induced unawareness, I wander, gibbering from my nursing home room with my blouse unbuttoned, my hair standing on end, and boogers bristling from my nose? Does my lack of awareness render me less dignified, or do I just seem less dignified to those who are more aware of my appearance or behavior than I am? If I even think about my dignity, I probably feel perfectly dignified.

The thought of being unaware and unwitting is embarrassing for me. But embarrassment or even sadness at seeing my loved one compromised by unawareness of his appearance, demeanor, bodily function, or mental acuity is distinct from my loved one's perception of his own dignity. The embarrassment and sadness are my own.

If we are supported in our "undignified" circumstances by loving, accepting people who do not perceive that we have lost our dignity— people who do not reflect to us by their own embarrassment, condescension, or pity that they believe we have lost our dignity—we can more easily find the inner strength to surmount the indignities of old age, ill health, or any of life's other "undignified" hurdles. At times our "undignified" process may be painful for others to watch, but it is, after all, *our* process.

My feelings regarding the "loss of dignity" haven't changed, but my thoughts on the subject have crystallized. So when I next hear the familiar, whispered "Oh how sad, so-and-so has lost his dignity," my response will probably be, "If you think he has lost his dignity, you are in an ideal position to return it to him."

Perhaps the challenges to dignity, which David and many of us will face at life's end, provide the ultimate opportunity for claiming rather than losing our essential dignity. By my definition, throughout the course of his tribulation, David has claimed extraordinary dignity.

Sweet Surprises

There have been many discouraging days when I see little evidence that David recognizes me. David now rarely remembers that Free-land, Michigan, is his birthplace; he typically does not distinguish between wife, daughter, son, and friend; and certainly he does not remember shared experiences. Other days, I believe he knows who I am but doesn't seem to care that I've come. I leave Willowglen asking myself the nagging question: *Does my presence still hold value for David?* One fleeting moment supplies the answer.

David's hand tremors have worsened, and I feed him whenever I visit at mealtime. I sit on his right side, out of his line of vision—*not* face-to-face as if feeding a baby. Without words, we have fallen into a routine. He sets the pace, chewing one bite while I load his fork and leave it on his plate. When he's ready, he signals me with raised eyebrows and a quick thrust of his chin.

One evening, he doesn't even acknowledge my arrival. Throughout the meal he is somber and unresponsive. After his last bite, I put down the fork. Without turning his head to look at me, David reaches for my hand and firmly squeezes it. I return his pressure. Still holding my hand, he faces me, smiles broadly, and gives me a long, fluttery wink.

In the days ahead, David may be unable to offer even these simple indicators that my gestures in his direction are meaningful to him. My challenge will be to remember the fluttery winks, to remain constant, regardless of what David can or cannot tell me.

IT IS 7 P.M. WHEN I KNOCK on the door of David's room. Hearing agitated voices on the other side, I enter without invitation. Stifling heat envelops me—heat so oppressive it would make anyone snarly. A caregiver stands by David's bed urging him to do something. She speaks in a thick accent even I can't understand.

Judging by the expression on David's face, there is no crisis in progress, just two wills clashing. David, in his underwear, is not exactly lying on his bed. Teetering on his side, his upper body clings to the edge of the bed; his legs, akimbo, extend limply to the floor. To maintain this gravity-defying position under the best of circumstances would be impressive. David's tenacity is especially noteworthy considering the heat, the fact that he is under duress from a caregiver whose mysterious agenda he is resisting, and he is simultaneously attempting to feign sleep during the lapses between his spirited retorts.

Catching my signal that I'll relieve her, the caregiver nods and silently retreats. I move to the side of the bed. David, still perilously draped on the edge, is inert except for his eyelids that twitch involuntarily from the strain of his charade.

Gently laying a hand on his shoulder I inquire, "Hey, David, what's going on?"

"Leave me the hell alone!" he bellows explosively.

"David, I don't think you even know who you're yelling at."

Tentatively, he lets his eyes flicker open to a squint. "Oh hello, Darling! Where did you come from?" he asks, grinning, as he props himself up on one elbow.

His greeting catches me off guard. It's been many weeks since David welcomed me so warmly and with such verbal clarity. I raise the windows a crack, help David into a bathrobe, and refresh him with a glass of water before we settle in to an evening of togetherness.

For almost two hours, I pamper David with pedicure, manicure, and massage. He is relaxed.

As I begin to massage his neck and shoulders, David says softly, "Ummm ... hands with love inside."

"Oh, David, I'm glad my hands feel loving to you."

He does not respond, and for the next quarter of an hour, the only words spoken are my own, "How ya doin', David?" or "David, this muscle in your neck feels tight. Does it hurt?" or "I think I can hear you purring, David."

He simply smiles or nods his responses.

Knowing the extent to which David's verbal skills have deteriorated, I am startled when he breaks the silence with, "You make me more of what I want to be." Later, he surprises me again when he murmurs, "It's best when you're here."

The evening ends. David is in bed. I lie beside him, my arms around him, my cheek on his. "I'll be lonely when you leave," he whispers.

A LOVED ONE sails alone on the sea of dementia. We are not privileged to board his ship, to know all of his realities. But we can sail alongside, calling out reassurances of our love and presence. Though each of us sails alone, we are empowered to ease the loneliness for our loved one and ourselves when we find the courage to shift our longing from what *was* to what *is* still possible.

Despite years of believing in David's ability to stretch to his highest potential, despite my adamant conviction that he has more mental capacity than he is able to reveal, I would have readily bet against his ability to articulate such endearing sentiments as "Hands with love inside," "You make me more of what I want to be," "It's best when you're here," or "I'll be lonely when you leave." Once again, I am humbled. Apparently, even I am guilty of occasionally holding limited expectations of David. By now I should know that his limitations, although extensive, manifest erratically and inconsistently— they do not progress neatly, do not lend themselves to linear categorizing. Consequently, David's deficits never clearly define him.

He must never be discounted or dismissed. So my antenna will remain fixed in David's direction for as long as he continues to signal me with fleeting glints of light from his fading intellect. No, I will be attuned even beyond his signaling.

David Turns Ninety-six

In the days before David's ninety-sixth birthday, Terry and I have frequent conversations about what kind of celebration will be most enjoyable for him. As always, his steadfast former associates call to suggest that they bring a birthday cake and their good wishes to Willowglen. Terry and I are torn. If David happens to be having one of his good days when his friends arrive, he will be thrilled that they remembered his special day. However, David's days are now marked not only by confusion but, unpredictably, by anxiety, occasional belligerence, and an inability to verbalize. Although his friends can handle whatever he presents, our concern is for David. How will he feel if he fails to recognize his friends or is unable to express his appreciation of their kind gesture? Surely he will be embarrassed to find himself in the spotlight without the skills to behave graciously. We finally settle on bringing a birthday cake to share with the staff and residents of Meadow House, the group of people with whom he seems to feel most comfortable these days.

On B-Day, Terry and I arrive at Willowglen toward the end of the noon meal. All the Meadow House residents are still at their tables. Michael and David's granddaughter, Katie, join us. We sing "Happy Birthday," present the cake, and after plenty of shouted encouragement from revelers and three valiant puffs from David, he extinguishes his ten candles: one candle for each of his nine decades completed, one candle for passing the halfway mark of his tenth decade. Although not exuberant, David is obviously pleased with all the attention. From his cell phone Michael calls Sissy at her office in New York. David seems to have a sense of who Sissy is, and a brief visit with her heightens his festive mood.

After thirty minutes, the cake-sated, party-weary residents of Meadow House are beginning to drift away in various directions. Michael and Katie have left, and Terry and I go with David to his room to open birthday cards and a few small gifts: handkerchiefs, a new belt, a box of candy. Although he repeatedly asks why he's receiving gifts, David tears into his presents with a child's gusto and exclaims happily over their contents. He stuffs one of the handkerchiefs into the breast pocket of his sport coat, puts on his new belt, and fills his pockets with candy. Flowers from Sissy have arrived earlier in the day. David points to them at least a dozen times, questioning where they came from and is repeatedly pleased with the answer that they are a birthday present from Sissy.

By midafternoon, David is mellow and drowsy. Without fanfare we kiss him good-bye and leave him relaxed and nodding in his chair.

A Broader Resolve

Five days have passed since David's birthday. Terry and I arrive for a visit. A large group of residents is in the dining room of Meadow House where they have been participating (in varying degrees) in a pizza-baking project. Most residents, David among them, are sitting in chairs arranged around the perimeter of the dining room, waiting for the pizza to materialize.

David shows no sign of recognition as we approach him. He is courteous but impersonal when we greet him—vaguely pleasant, as if, "I can tell I should know you, but I honestly don't know who you are." He shrugs off our strokes of affection.

There are no seats for us near David. We suggest that the three of us go to his room so we can have a private visit.

He responds, "Why should I? What are you talking about? Leave me alone."

Thinking he may not want to miss his share of the pizza, we offer to take pizza to his room.

"This is nonsense," he snarls. "Just stop, will you! What do you want?"

Eventually David grudgingly agrees to go with us to his room, but his attitude is unchanged. Even his favorite snack, the grapes that Terry always brings when she visits, serves as an irritant.

"What am I supposed to do with these? I can't eat all of these. This is ridiculous."

After an hour of sullen resistance to our attentions, David begins to doze in his armchair. Without rousing him to say good-bye, we move toward the door and turn down the long hall outside of his room. At the end of the hall, we glance back at David's door. He is standing in the doorway watching us. We wave. He doesn't acknowledge us, and we continue toward the exit.

Over the years I have known David to exhibit surprising canniness. I wonder if he has shrewdly feigned sleep to rid himself of our company.

I FIND I NEED TO take a few emotional steps back. As I begin to distance myself from the events of the afternoon, I discover what may be David's perspective: He was content when we arrived. He didn't seem to recognize us. We insinuated ourselves into his activity and rearranged his agenda. It might have been better for him if we had said, "David, it's good to see you, but it looks like you're busy right now. We don't want to intrude, so we'll come back another time soon."

Had we respected him in this way, he might have agreed it was best for us to leave, or he might have had a shift in attitude that would have allowed him to participate with us. Either way, we would have empowered him. As it was, we treated him paternalistically; our actions told him we knew what was best for him, and he had no vote.

If we truly care about David and want what is best for him, why do we lock ourselves into behavior that is unrewarding for him and for us? I think back to my recent resolution to be attuned to David even beyond his signaling.

When I committed myself to being alert to his needs, I was thinking in more sentimental terms. I was imagining sweet-spirited David, sentient but unable to communicate. Beyond this possibility, I saw a time when he might not be sentient but still able to receive the warmth and support of human affection. Today's scenario presents a new twist: a communicative but irritable David who doesn't want support from two people he views, at least for the moment, as unwelcome outsiders. If we are dedicated to doing what is best for David, I believe we must listen to him, even to the point of accepting his negative protests, regardless of the energy we've invested in a visit, no matter how far we have traveled to be with him. Instead of focusing on our frustration at being spurned, we can be thankful that on this day, David is comfortable and content within his familiar environment.

Today, David did signal with a glint of light from his fading intellect. Eventually we received his signal, but our receiving was not in time to be of the greatest value to him. Now, my earlier resolve has broadened to encompass an intention to accept the possibility that David's needs may, at times, be better met by our absence rather than our presence. Setting aside our own egos in favor of supporting him (in whatever frame of mind we find him) will surely be liberating for all of us. And tomorrow is a new day—a day when David may welcome a visit.

An Improvised Vocabulary

David's language skills have deteriorated, but his drive to communicate and my eagerness to understand him and respond appropriately have not diminished. Unfortunately, my eagerness does not mean that I'm not often stymied.

Sometimes I can determine what a word means from its context, as when David frantically and repeatedly pats all of his pockets, murmuring distractedly, "My frible, my frible."

"David, are you looking for your billfold?"

"Yes, yes!" he answers anxiously.

"Oh, David, remember, you recently decided not to carry a bill-fold anymore. Too hard to keep track of. Now you just pay for everything once a month by check," I remind him.

He accepts this explanation, but soon he repeats the pat-down, and I repeat the explanation.

I have never heard David use the same invented word twice to refer to the same thing. One day, billfold is "frible," the next day (or hour or minute) it may be "mithra."

Too often, I resort to the timeworn "David, I'm sorry, I'm confused."

Usually, he laughs and gives me a nod or, on good days, his once-standard "Me too," indicating he is confused as well. He is no longer able to repeat or paraphrase what he said moments earlier, but he also doesn't remember he was trying to tell me anything, so he is not frustrated.

David's improvised vocabulary fascinates me, and I pay close attention, often writing down his impromptu ramblings. Sometimes my attentiveness is rewarded. Today is one of those times.

We've just returned from a haircut outing—the only outing we take these days. David is chattering in determined bursts of jargon, which, to my ears, sound nonsensical but intriguing. I'm listening carefully to see if I can catch a thread of meaning from his elaborate, multisyllabic miscellany of sound.

I have just volunteered, "David, you're ninety-six years old now. Your agenda is not as full as it once was. You're taking it easy for a change—a well-deserved break after a long and illustrious career."

David is frowning, shaking his head, protesting my statement in his own language. Abruptly, his expression changes. He is smiling as he begins to speak animatedly in words known only to him—maybe not even him. Interspersed among these alien-sounding words, delivered with earnest expression and inflection, are a few familiar words from our common language.

"Spreegaliss … burs … bursborin … uh … reremember … propa … pro … pro … propalicrity … um … um-ba-them-e-nal … now …

and then … shiffle … shaff … uh … uh … feckerd … bofod … I … made … a wave," David says, grinning, and looking at me expectantly.

From this bizarre conglomeration of verbiage, I patch together the phrase "Remember, now and then, I made a wave."

"David, did you say, 'Remember, now and then, I made a wave'?" I ask.

"Of course," he says matter-of-factly.

Does David want me to remember him after he is *gone*—to recall from time to time that he made a wave? Is he just casually asking me to reminisce with him *at this moment*—to remember that "now and then," in his lifetime, he made a wave, stirred things up, had an impact? The nuance may not matter to David. Either way, I'm caught off guard.

"David you have *definitely* made a wave. In fact, over the years, you've made many waves, large and small—waves that have made a difference in people's lives—wonderful waves that have changed the city of Denver," I manage to squeak out as emotion tightens my throat.

Still smiling, David nods vigorously and responds, "Yes … right … really?"

I wonder what has triggered this moment of seeming clarity. Perhaps an actual memory of some past accomplishment filtered through, or more simply the sense that we have come close to a real conversation.

Following the pattern of all our exchanges these days, this conversation leaves me with more questions than answers. Foremost, I wonder if, in spite of David's come-and-go self-awareness, he is still trying to integrate who he is now with who he once was—still trying to hang on to his essential self. And I wonder if my responses are everything he needs them to be.

On David-Time

The adrenaline-producing pace of life in the twenty-first century—a pace defined by TV, radio, traffic, headlines, deadlines, too many responsibilities, and countless preoccupations—is not in sync with the rhythms of one who is in the late stages of dementia. David now lives in a dimension where time is irrelevant. When I visit him, I try to experience as much of his timeless reality as I can. It has become my habit, as I walk from the parking lot to the door of Willowglen, to consciously ratchet down my twenty-first century energy by breathing deeply and focusing exclusively on the moment at hand. I do this not to brace myself for what I'll encounter on the other side of the door, but to fully open myself to *whatever* awaits me.

To assure my focus, I have devised something of a mantra:

> There's only one place I can be at this moment,
> I give myself over to being here only.

ONE DAY I ARRIVE to find David in a compromising predicament. I hear and smell the challenge before I see it. David's unmistakable voice is raised in an emphatically repeated, "Leave me alone, damn it," and the stench of a call from nature that went unanswered permeates the corridor leading to Meadow House.

I find David in a standoff with a caregiver who is trying to pull him toward his room while futilely fanning the air and telegraphing her revulsion. Stepping in front of this unfortunate duo, I kneel down in front of David, putting myself in his line of vision so we can make eye contact and he can see that I'm smiling.

"Hey David," I begin. "I'm here to help you."

"Who the hell are you?" he growls.

"I'm Marilyn, and we're on our way to your room so you can clean up." Lightly, nonthreateningly, I place my hand on his lower leg and for two silent seconds we just look at each other.

I stand up, entwine my arm with his and continue chatting as we move down the hall. The relieved caregiver mouths, "Thank you," and goes in another direction.

"I see the cut on your forehead is healing nicely ... I'm always amazed at how fast you heal, David ... Have you been outside today?

The sun is bright, but a nippy fall breeze is blowing ... almost too brisk for strolling outside ..."

Maybe I'm taking unfair advantage by bombarding David with non sequiturs, but a distraction seems in order.

In David's room we begin the forty-five-minute clean-up process—peeling off the saturated clothes, showering, washing the overflow out of David's shoes. Between his bursts of incoherent chatter we sing songs from other eras: "Side by Side," "Always," "The Sidewalks of New York," "If I Loved You." Occasionally David plugs in a word, but mostly he contributes by booming out the tune—operatically, complete with tremolos—through lips rounded into a wide-open "O." He still remembers the tune of every song we "sing."

David is nearly reassembled. He is sitting in a chair, and I am kneeling on the floor putting his socks on, looking up into his face.

Clearly and directly, David says, "Hi, Doll, we're havin' fun now."

This is the only lucid thing he says to me for the rest of the afternoon.

I DON'T ENJOY dealing with an old man's diarrhea any more than the next person, but I can truthfully say that since supporting David is my goal, I view even the diarrhea challenges as just another way to be with David, to meet him wherever he finds himself, and to invest in our relationship. Arriving at this perspective has been an evolutionary process. It seems my evolution has taken about as long as David's decline, but I have actually come to believe that a forty-five-minute clean-up session is a more fulfilling way to spend our time than sitting formally side by side, frustrating ourselves by trying to carry on a meaningful conversation. So much better to be working together on a project—laughing, singing, touching, and moving toward a common goal.

From a broader perspective, I have realized a life-changing benefit as a result of my years with David. This benefit is my increased ability to cope with the derailments that feel large on the track of my life. Now I worry little about the number of days allotted to me. Death is inevitable, but as it turns out, life is inevitable too. Through David, I have learned the importance of rooting myself in present time … then living.

Every one of us is riding steadily into the sunset. I have been privileged to be David's traveling "pardner"—riding with him for many years, seeing twilight through his eyes.

Truth … Not Pity

What? Pity?
You should save *that* for another.
The *truth* is what I really need from you.
Oh yes … your touch,
A moment of shared laughter;
How sweet these are,
'Til now, I never knew.

—M. M., 1999

Reflections on a Final Parting

Adventure, meaningful relationship, and life lessons were the hallmarks of my time with David Touff. As David and I traveled together, I saw first hand that people tend to underestimate the capacities of those who have dementia. David demonstrated that a man losing his brilliant mind is still capable of establishing a fulfilling relationship and joyously engaging in his life for years after he began to exhibit the symptoms of dementia. David's story encourages us to seek new perspectives and offers a heartening contrast to more limiting approaches to memory loss. My simple receptiveness to David and his circumstances enabled me to learn some of my most valuable life lessons, caused me to reevaluate my view of an individual's worth, and brought me into closer alignment with my own humanity.

After eight years of friendship with David, the day I simultaneously longed for and dreaded seemed imminent. David was 97, and countless times over the years had said, "People aren't supposed to live this long! How the hell does a guy get out of here?"

While David wistfully contemplated his mortality, I was deeply saddened by the thought of life without him. At least "the long goodbye" allowed me ample time to say it and adjust to new realities. I also found comfort in my belief that the stimulation of our adventures had slowed the progress of David's dementia and enhanced his latter years.

Despite his previous "how-to-get-out-of-here" queries, during David's final months, he boomeranged back from various infections, massive seizures, and punishing falls that sent him to the emergency room for elaborate suturing. His ironclad will to live mystified me, and I could not imagine how or when he would leave us.

Then came a shift. In the space of several days, David's appetite waned, his motor skills deteriorated, he slept more, and his drastically-diminished cognition faded further. That mysterious catalyst—precursor of life's end—was evidently at work. Still David resisted death with the same purposeful intensity that had defined his life.

Having been with David on Sunday and Monday, I had not planned to visit him on Tuesday. But shortly after five o'clock on Tuesday evening, I was working at my desk when I felt an unexpected urge to drive twenty miles through rain and rush-hour traffic to be with my friend. I had no sense that haste was imperative—only a single-minded intention to move steadily in David's direction.

As I entered Willowglen, I met Michael. He said he was going out for some dinner and would see me later.

David was in bed; his eyes were open and fixed on the ceiling; his breathing was rhythmic—more deliberate than labored. Prepared to stay indefinitely, I lay down beside him.

Moments later, Michael returned. "I couldn't leave without saying a proper goodbye to you," he offered.

Pulling a chair close to the bed, he sat down and took his father's hand. We spoke little, and David seemed unaware of our presence, yet soon the three of us fell into a silent union—a meditation guided by the steady meter of David's breathing. We had been together only minutes when David raised his head from the pillow, pushed firmly against our supporting hands with his own, then sank back to restfulness. He closed his eyes, took two more breaths, and settled easily into eternity. The thought flashed: *It came so quickly!* Yet David had lived more than a decade in mental disarray.

Initially I was jubilant. David had found his way "out of here," and Michael and I, having managed to coalesce in an improbable window of opportunity, were privileged to be present for the end of David's remarkable life.

My elation was fleeting. With the finality of death came a heavy melancholy, then a peculiar discord as I vacillated between feeling bereft and thrilled. I had lost my cherished friend, but he had been released from a tormenting bondage. For David I felt only joy—for myself, only sadness.

Reflecting on the ebbing moments of David's life, I realize I have been left with a penetrating sense that I participated in something sacred. Those few hallowed minutes at the end of David's life informed my view of death—demystified the dying process, and integrated death harmoniously into life's circle—a final lesson from David.

Appendix A

Activities

As David's dementia progresses I realize I can no longer create adventures for him. I need to narrow my focus and create simple activities.

Although I try to devise a wide variety of activities for David, I realize that diversity in our choices of activities is more for my benefit than for his. David doesn't remember an activity from one hour to the next. I need variety to prevent my own boredom—to help me maintain genuine enthusiasm during our time together.

When creating diversions for David, I follow one guiding principle: Have a plan, but don't become wedded to a goal. A plan always gets us up and moving in a direction. A goal often proves to be too confining and frustrating. By tuning in to the realities and needs of the moment with David, I have gradually learned to let go of my own expectations for an activity. When I'm with David, I constantly remind myself, "My only purpose is to facilitate David's joy and contentment as he participates *in his own way.*"

Following are activities that are scattered throughout the book. I list them here for readers' convenience and as springboards to stimulate ideas for other activities. My goal when creating an activity is not merely to fill time but to give David an opportunity to reestablish his sense of himself and his connection to life's mainstream.

- ATM Machine—An activity with a built-in accomplishment that doesn't require leaving the car! The mysterious and high-tech quality of drive-through banking creates a certain intrigue and excitement for David.
- Books—For David, well-chosen books are an activity mainstay. Some of his favorites are picture books, books of quotations such as *Bartlett's Familiar Quotations,* and books of facts such as *Ripley's*

Believe-It-Or-Not and *The Guinness Book of World Records*. Basic books on any subject of particular interest to the individual work well. The children's section of the library can be a great resource for basic books about history, geography, poetry, etc.

- Car Wash—A drive-through car wash provides a sense of accomplishment and the thrill of adventure. The accomplishment aspect is always heightened when I express my appreciation to David; for example, "Thank you, David, for coming with me to wash the car. It is great to have your company, and it's a pleasure to finally have a clean car!"

- Catalogs—Looking at mail order catalogs together is a satisfying pastime—a form of window-shopping. This activity requires no specific memory or reference to time. The pictures are self-evident, will stimulate whatever memory is available to the viewer, and serve as topics for conversation. The nature of the activity also creates physical closeness. Often, David's contentment comes not from the activity so much as from my willingness to be focused on and physically close to him.

- Crossword Puzzles and Other Word Games—As with catalogs, the enjoyment of puzzles and games requires no specific memory or reference to time. However, one must choose puzzles and games with the individual in mind. Activities that are too elementary or too advanced are frustrating.

- Dialoguing—Generating and maintaining conversation with one who has dementia can be challenging. A number of books offer questions that can trigger conversation. One such title is *To Our Children's Children*, Bob Greene (Doubleday, New York, 1993), and *The Book of Questions*, Gregory Stock, Ph.D. (Workman Publishing, New York, 1985, 1987). This activity provides the physical closeness and individual focus that David craves.

- Everyday Life Flow—In my home, I included David in as many household activities as possible: sorting clothes for the laundry, emptying the bedroom wastebaskets, opening the shades and turning off the front porch lights in the morning, watering the houseplants, putting newspapers in the recycle bin, etc. If there are mishaps in the process, I view them as custom-made, everyday, life-flow activities.

- Family Pictures—David never tires of looking at family pictures. This is an opportunity to finally sort through the shoe boxes of photos and organize them into albums.
- Garage Sales—David thoroughly enjoys seeing what other people have spent their money on and what they are eager to sell. Maybe this comes from his years as a retailer and is not universally intriguing. David was thrilled with his purchase of a ten-cent coffee mug. For years he used the mug every morning until I accidentally broke it.
- Grocery Shopping—This activity provides needed exercise and mental stimulation.
- Library Browsing—This is another destination, and an opportunity to see a broad spectrum of people. David likes to people-watch, especially children. He also seems to enjoy the congenial, library hustle-bustle. Sometimes he even looks at the books! This is an activity that serves us both, because I can do my own browsing as long as David is enjoying himself.
- Rides—The benefit of this activity is the movement and the scenery. As David's dementia progresses, my car is the only way to travel. Public transportation is no longer a good option.
- Singing—Whether with the radio, with old movie soundtracks, or with a video musical, singing offers the benefit of participation and the familiarity of old favorites. Singing from songbooks of oldies is great fun, even without accompaniment.
- Treats—Venturing out for a simple hamburger is a thrill for David. Pie and coffee, ice cream cones, fresh baked goods from the bakery down the street—pursuing these small pleasures provides a destination and adds importance to a day.

PEOPLE WITH DEMENTIA take many of their emotional cues from others, so I suggest to David only activities for which I myself have genuine enthusiasm. He rarely cares whether we do activity A or B, but he picks up on my attitude about an activity and enjoys the activity, or not, accordingly.

Appendix B

Finding the Right Home

If there is truth in the statement "A house is not a home without love," how much truer this maxim is for those who have dementia. It was in the spirit of wanting love and nurturing for David that Terry and I looked for a place that would be a *home* for David. Following are the guidelines that evolved as we visited various facilities:

- Activities—Is there a regular and well-implemented schedule of activities for the residents, including an art, movement, and music program that allows them to sing along, not just be entertained?
- Balanced Competency Levels—I believe that those residents who are in the final and extremely dysfunctional stages of dementia (catatonic or comatose), or those who are aggressive and/or disruptive to other residents, should be accommodated separately. I also believe that residents who are less functional—still aware and nonthreatening—benefit tremendously from association with residents who are *more* functional. However, I have observed that when higher-functioning residents are in the minority, they become demoralized. Exceptions to this observation (sexist though it may sound) are the nurturing female residents who cast themselves in the role of caregivers.
- Demeanor of Residents—Are residents alert and responsive, appropriate to their stages of dementia? Does the demeanor of the general population seem compatible with the demeanor of your loved one?
- Director with Whom You Feel Comfortable—You must have a sense of ease and rapport with the on-site facility director. He/she must have good communication skills, be accountable, and be willing to follow through in solving problems. Problems *will* arise, and you will need more than a pretty face at the helm.

- Environment—Are the surroundings aesthetically pleasing and well maintained?
- Food—Are the meals and snacks well balanced, tasty, and attractively presented?
- Friendliness—Is there a nurturing, congenial attitude, free from condescension, toward residents?
- General Atmosphere—Is the atmosphere serene, positive, and hopeful? Look at the faces of the staff, especially caregivers, for eye contact, warmth, welcoming smiles. Staff members tend to be on their best behavior in the presence of visitors. If you object to what you see, either in the manner you yourself are received or in the attitude toward residents, you should wonder if the situation is worse when there are no visiting "witnesses." Look for rapport among staff members. A warm rapport among staff members filters down to the resident population.
- Light—Is there natural and plentiful light?
- Location—Look first at nursing homes in your area. The farther you are from the facility, the more burdensome will be the visiting and the less likely you will be to visit regularly.
- Music—Is there music playing? The right kind of music adds a soothing influence and a sense of life and animation. But the volume of the music should not dominate the environment.
- Ratios—Are there adequate staff-to-resident ratios (six or seven residents to each caregiver)?
- Respect—Is there demonstrated respect for the residents as feeling human beings, not as a subhuman population to be managed? Staff should not talk in the presence of residents as if residents were not present.
- Security—Is the indoor and outdoor security adequate to ensure that residents do not wander away?
- Spaces (Indoor)—Are the indoor spaces large enough for comfortable movement and diversion when the weather is inclement?
- Spaces (Outdoor)—Are the outdoor spaces for walking and being active large enough to accommodate the residential population?

- Staff—Is the entire staff well trained and competent?
- Tranquilizers—Determine that there is no general use of tranquilizers to ensure a malleable population.
- Visiting for Purposes of Evaluation—Visit a minimum of three facilities. No facility is perfect. Once you place your loved one, you will see flaws, even in the best facility. When the flaws become evident, doubt and guilt may enter your mind. You will be comforted by remembering where you *didn't* place your loved one, and that you *did* make a sincere effort to find the best facility possible. Visiting several facilities in advance of placement is easier on all concerned than relocating your loved one after he/she has entered a facility.

Trust your instincts!

Appendix C

Resources

"If you've met one person with Alzheimer's disease,
you've met just one person with Alzheimer's disease."*
—David Troxel, Executive Director
Alzheimer's Association, Santa Barbara Chapter

Recognizing that dementia of any type does not erase a person's individuality is fundamental to creating the best possible program of care and support for one who has dementia. There is no one-size-fits-all program, and many resources that did not exist until recently, are now available for designing individualized care.

Because Alzheimer's/dementia has become something of an epidemic, support resources are expanding in proportion to the prevalence of the disease. This evolution is so rapid that resources I identified only months ago are already outdated. However, the Alzheimer's Association is always in the vanguard of everything related to Alzheimer's/dementia, and I strongly recommend that the association be the first resource readers investigate.

The Alzheimer's Association national information number is 800-272-3900. The Alzheimer's Association website is: www.alz.org. Local chapters are listed in the phone book under "Alzheimer's Association." They will send an information packet—my packet arrived twenty-four hours after I called.

There are dozens of chapters of the National Alzheimer's Association, many chapters in every state. The resources and compassionate support that are available through this remarkable organization are

---

*Virginia Bell and David Troxel, *The Best Friends Approach to Alzheimer's Care*, Baltimore: Health Professions Press, 1999. Reprinted with permission.

outstanding. Many of the volunteers have had firsthand experience with Alzheimer's in their families. Speaking with someone who understands is tremendously reassuring.

Alzheimer's Association's services include:

- Community Resources—A directory of programs in your area for respite or day care
- Counseling
- Family Education
- Helpline
- Library—Alzheimer's-related books, tapes, and videos
- Special Seminars—Instruction for caregivers
- Support Groups

Appendix D

An Alzheimer's Disease Bill of Rights

Every person diagnosed with Alzheimer's disease or a related disorder deserves:

- To be informed of one's diagnosis
- To have appropriate, ongoing medical care
- To be productive in work and play as long as possible
- To be treated like an adult, not a child
- To have expressed feelings taken seriously
- To be free from psychotropic medications if at all possible
- To live in a safe, structured, and predictable environment
- To enjoy meaningful activities that fill each day
- To be out-of-doors on a regular basis
- To have physical contact including hugging, caressing, and hand-holding
- To be with people who know one's life story, including cultural and religious traditions
- To be cared for by individuals well-trained in dementia care*

(*Virginia Bell and David Troxel, *The Best Friends Approach to Alzheimer's Care*, Baltimore: Health Professions Press, 1999. Reprinted with permission.)

IT IS MY STRONG BELIEF that if we neglect to employ the Alzheimer's Disease Bill of Rights, we fail one who has dementia in two ways: we diminish the quality of his days and we hasten the progress of his decline. Treated with disrespect and given little hope, he will rapidly fulfill our lowest expectations of him. But a caregiver's respect helps the person who has dementia to believe in his abilities and inspires him to continually stretch to his highest level of competency. Perhaps this respectful process even slows the rate of his deterioration.

Appendix E

Dance Steps for Caregivers

The "steps" below are also woven throughout the book. I have brought them together here for easy reference:

1. Truthfulness
   - In public, spare your friend and others the embarrassment of absolute truthfulness.
   - In private, patiently and lovingly tell your friend even the hardest truths.
2. Straight Talk
   - When you don't understand, say so. Saying you're confused, "levels the playing field."
   - When talking with your friend, use his name frequently to anchor him to the conversation and to remind him that the two of you have a relationship.
   - Repeat the subject of a conversation frequently to refresh your friend's memory and to help him maintain his focus.
   - Avoid using pronouns like he, she, him, her, they, them, it. Refer specifically, by name, to the person, place or thing you are talking about.
   - Use a conversational "time-out" or a change of subject to break the cycle of an obsessive verbal "loop." To avoid confusion, tell your friend what you're doing. For Example, "David, I'm going to stop talking for a few minutes and just enjoy this wonderful food." Or, "David, let's change the subject for a moment."
   - Talk daily with your friend about his own history.
3. Practicalities
   - Careful grooming is essential for your friend's morale. It also affects how the world responds to him. He deserves your support in presenting himself as attractively as possible so others will respond to him as positively as possible.

- Offer choices to your friend only when you can comfortably accept what he chooses.
- Choose activities that interest *you*, and your friend will likely reflect your enthusiasm.

4. Chosen Perspectives
   - You choose your perspective—an invaluable thing to remember in dark hours.
   - Give your friend credit for knowing more than he is capable of expressing. He probably does know more. If he doesn't, what's the harm?
   - Your friend is less mentally and emotionally flexible than you are. Try to be flexible for both of you.
   - Your friend needs your acceptance and willingness to participate with him exactly as he is at any given moment.
   - You have no "lessons" to teach. Your friend is beyond lessons. Besides, you are the student.
   - See yourself in your friend. Discovering your common humanity will open your heart to him. An open heart creates the best outcome.
   - Your friend won't hold your mistakes against you for long. Try to be equally forgiving.
   - Give up lofty goals. Look for meaning in the moment.
   - Try laughing before crying.
   - When laughing fails, cry … hard.

(Note: To avoid the he/she gender tangle, and because *Dancing on Quicksand* is about David, I used "he" exclusively in the "steps" above.)